Pocket Guides for Gynaecologists

Editors: Thomas Römer, Andreas D. Ebert

W0037948

Thomas Römer

Operative Hysteroscopy

A Practical Guide

2nd Edition

DE GRUYTER

Professor Dr. med. Thomas Römer
Evangelisches Krankenhaus
Köln-Weyertal gGmbH
Weyertal 76
50931 Köln
Email: Thomas.Roemer@EVK-Koeln.de
Translated by Dr. Christina Römer, Cologne.

This book contains 96 figures and 34 tables.

The book series Gynaecological Pocket Guides was founded by Prof. Dr. med. Wolfgang Straube, Rostock and Prof. Dr. Thomas Römer, Köln.

ISBN 978-3-11-022499-3
e-ISBN 978-3-11-022500-6

Library of Congress Cataloging-in-Publication Data

A CIP catalogue record for this book is available from the Library of Congress.

Bibliographic information published by the Deutsche Nationalbibliothek

The Deutsche Nationalbibliothek lists this publication in the Deutsche Nationalbibliografie; detailed bibliographic data are available in the Internet at http://dnb.d-nb.de.

Typesetting and printing: Beltz Bad Langensalza GmbH, Bad Langensalza

Printed in Germany
www.degruyter.com

Preface

The new edition of "Operative Hysteroscopy" again complements the 2nd edition of "Diagnostic Hysteroscopy. A Practical Guide", which was published in February 2010.

This pocket guide for gynaecologists should present the newcomer to operative hysteroscopy with a survey of the indications, contraindications and potential complications. Moreover, this pocket guide could be of use for informing and advising the patients.

In the last few years the operative hysteroscopy has become a standard method, also due to the latest technical innovations.

By the establishment of the bipolar technology in operative hysteroscopy the rate of complications might continue to decline. This new aspect is especially considered. Additionally, alternative methods to the endometrial ablation are presented and integrated into the range of therapies.

In a separate chapter special cases of the operative hysteroscopy are presented. A lot of pictures and tables underline the pocket guide character of this publication.

I would like to thank Dr. Bischoff, head of the Department of Anaesthetics and Intensive Care at the Academic Hospital Cologne-Weyertal for his support with the chapter on complications.

Special thanks to Ms Timm for typing the manuscript. I would also like to thank the publishing house for a long-term co-operation, special thanks are extended to Ms. Dr. Kowalski, who has always given her best attention to the project.

The company Karl Storz Ltd, especially Dr. h.c. Sibyll Storz, deserve a special gratitude for a consistent promotion of our endoscopic pocket guides.

I hope that this pocket guide contributes to a further propagation of the operative hysteroscopy.

Cologne, August 2011 Prof. Dr. med. Thomas Römer

Contents

Abbreviations

ACOG	American College of Obstetricians and Gynaecologists
CRP	C-reactive protein
ET	estrogen therapy
ESGE	European Society of Gynaecological Endoscopy
EUP	extrauterine pregnancy
Hb	haemoglobin
HF	high frequency
HT	hormone therapy
HSG	hysterosalpingography
IUA	intrauterine adhesions
IUD	intrauterine device
IUS	intrauterine system
LASH	laparoscopic supracervical hysterectomy
LAVH	laparoscopically assisted vaginal hysterectomy
MRI	magnet resonance imaging
OR	odds ratio
TLH	total laparoscopic hysterectomy
TUR	transurethral resection
W	Watt

1 Introduction

After the diagnostic hysteroscopy has been increasingly established as a standard method at hospitals and in gynaecological practices in the last few years, therapeutic interventions are gaining in importance, too. Compared with the diagnostic hysteroscopy, the operative hysteroscopy requires a considerably higher effort with regard to the technical equipment as well as the staff requirements.

In the therapy of infertility the operative hysteroscopy has completely replaced conventional techniques, which in most of the cases required a laparotomy. This applies to the treatment of the uterus septus, of intrauterine adhesions and submucous myomas. With bleeding disorders, which cannot be conservatively treated, hysteroscopic surgeries such as polyp – or myoma resection or the endometrial ablation, constitute alternative, organ-retaining methods of treatment.

Advantages of these endoscopic techniques are a minimal discomfort for the patient and the retaining of the organ. However, the operative hysteroscopy presents a lot of challenges for the surgeon since specific complications which require a wide knowledge of the safety aspects of the method may occur.

The present pocket book is meant to be a guide and a help for the acquisition of the techniques of operative hysteroscopy. It can, however, only support the absolutely necessary practical training.

With exact indications and with consideration of all safety aspects, the operative hysteroscopy is enrichment for the operative gynaecology.

2 Indications for operative hysteroscopy

With infertility:
- septum dissection with uterus subseptus/septus
- intrauterine adhesiolysis with adhesions grades III–IV/ESGE
- myoma resection

With bleeding disorders:
- myoma resection
- polyp resection
- endometrial ablation/endometrial resection

Special indications:
- resection of residual placenta
- opening or coagulation of a haematometra in the rudimentary uterine horn

3 Instrumentation and technical equipment

Necessary basic equipment for operative hysteroscopy:
- hysteroresectoscope with matching electrode and 12 degree angle lenses
- light source with cable
- Hysteromat with inflow and outflow tube
- distending medium
- video camera
- high frequency unit

Hysteroresectoscope

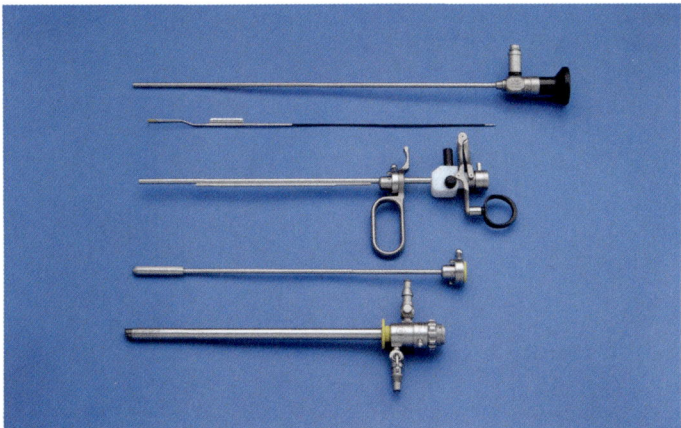

Fig. 3.1: Parts of the hysteroresectoscope:
- 12°-lenses
- electrode
- monopolar resectoscope
- obturator
- outer and inner sheath with inflow and outflow tubes for the distending medium

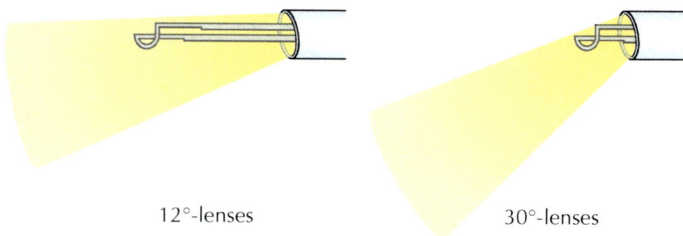

12°-lenses   30°-lenses

Fig. 3.2: Different perspectives with the 12° and 30°-lenses.
12°-lenses: electrode during the whole cutting and coagulation process in view
30°-lenses: electrode partially out of view

Note: For electrosurgical interventions 12°-angle lenses are recommended.

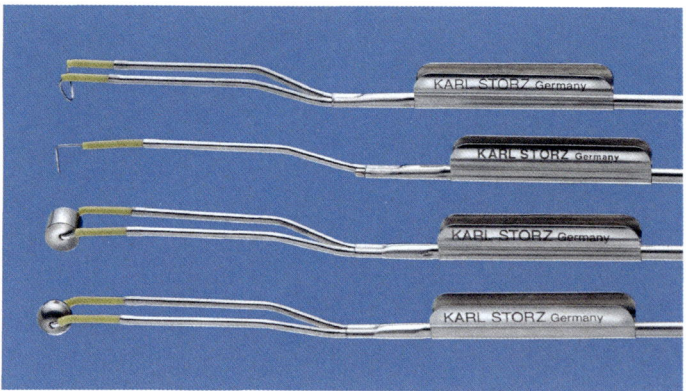

Fig. 3.3: Electrodes for the monopolar resectoscope.
- resection loop
- resection/dissection needle
- roller-bare
- roller-ball

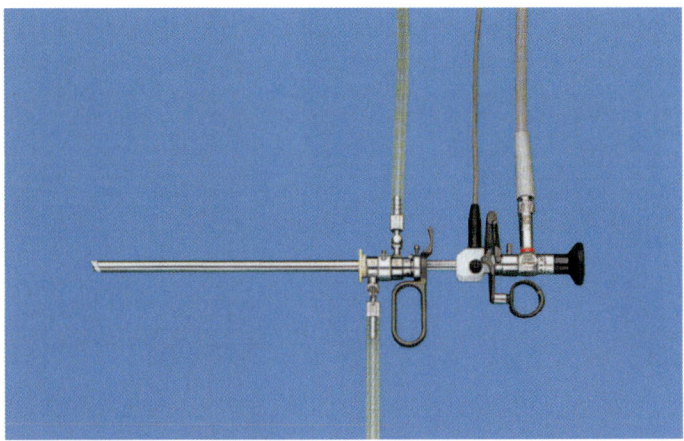

Fig. 3.4: Monopolar hysteroresectoscope (passive element), assembled, with all connections.
On the top from left to right:
- inflow tube for the distending medium
- connection of the high frequency unit Autocon II 400
- connection of the light cable
bottom:
- outflow tube for the distending medium

Electrodes in non-activated position:
- Advantage of the passive element: increased safety because during rotation the electrode is positioned in the sheath without
- Advantage of the active element: active movement during resection

Note: If possible, keep using the same hysteroresectoscope (passive or active element) – best training effect!

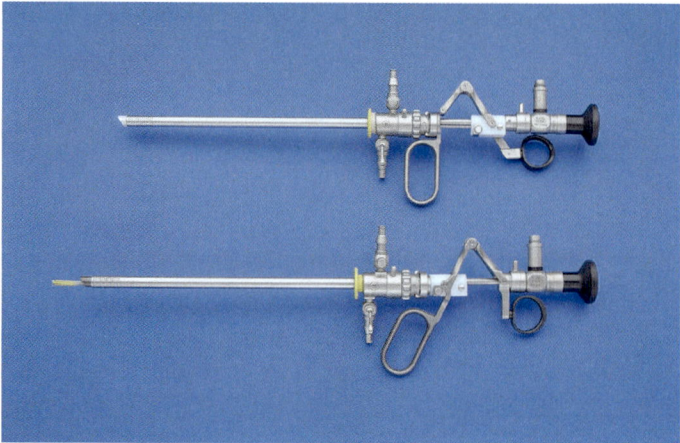

Fig. 3.5: Types of hysteroresectoscopes.
top: passive element
bottom: active element

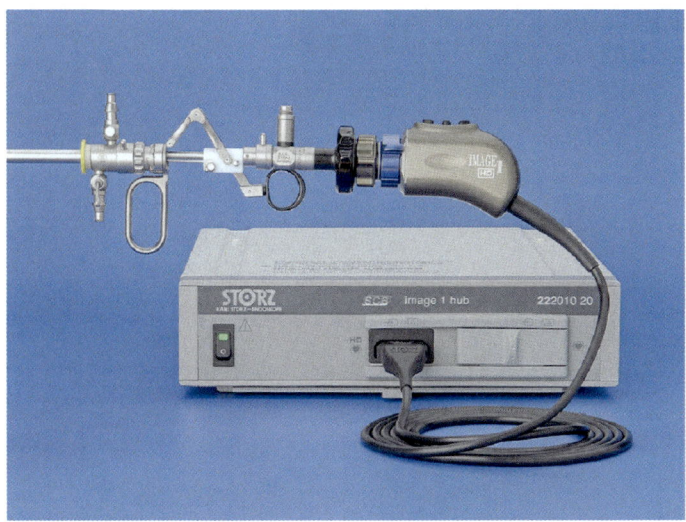

Fig. 3.6: Hysteroscope with video camera (Image 1/HD) and control gear.

Note: The application of HD-camera technology results in better pictures and clearer contours and thus increases the comfort for the surgeon as well as the safety for the patient during surgery.

HAMOU hysteromat

- pressure preselection
  recommendation: 150mm/Hg
  – sufficient pressure for distension of the cavity
- flow preselection
  recommendation: 200 ml/min
  – sufficient flow for the distension of the cavity and for irrigation
- passive fluid outflow by pressing the outflow tap **without** any additional generation of a vacuum

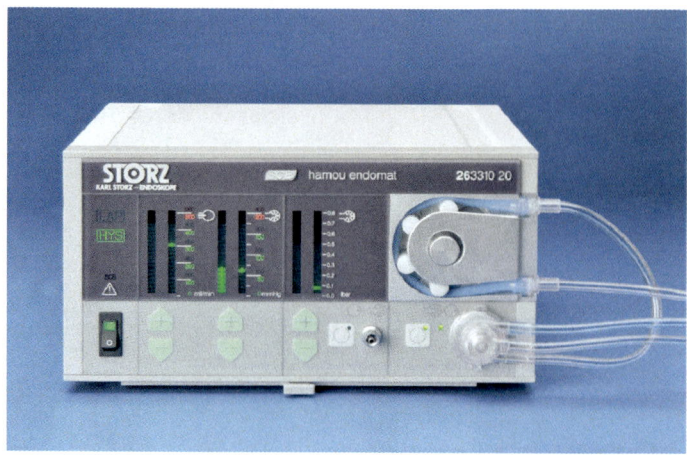

Fig. 3.7: Hysteromat with tubes connected to the roller pump.

Preselection
Left: preselect flow in ml/min to 200
Middle: preselect pressure in mm/Hg to 150
Right: not needed for vacuum extraction since a passive out-
         flow of the distending   medium is better

Note: With an active vacuum extraction the perforations of the hysteroscope may be blocked and thus obstruct the outflow and limit the intraoperative view.

Fig. 3.8: Complete video equipment (video tower) *from top to* ▶
bottom:
• monitor with a second rotatable monitor
• light source with camera control gear
• HAMOU endomat, endoflator
• second light source with second camera control gear
• AIDA documentation system and morcellator control gear
• Autocon II 400 (high frequency unit) High frequency unit

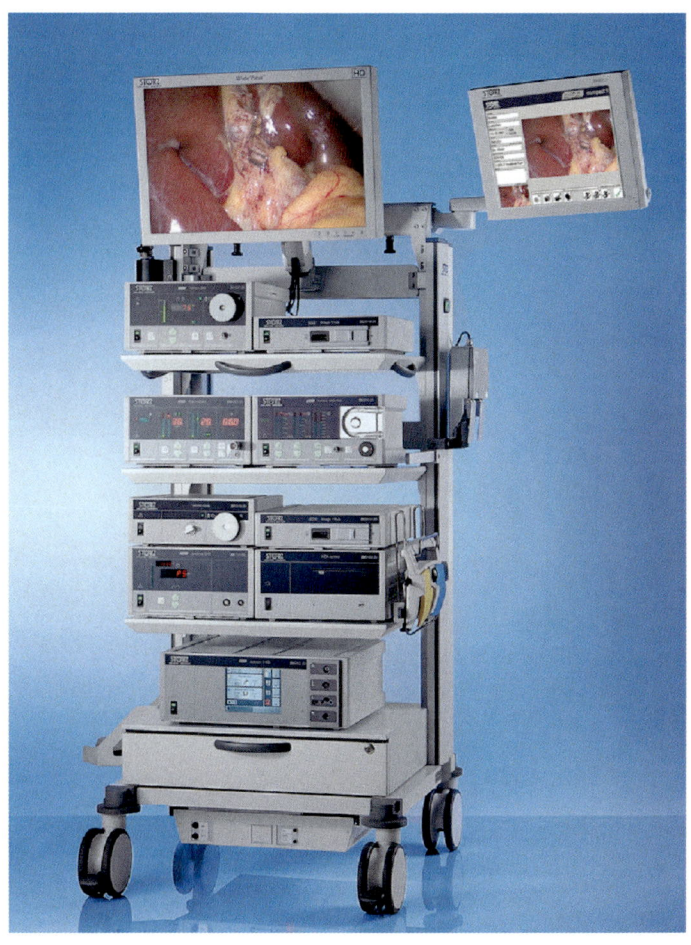

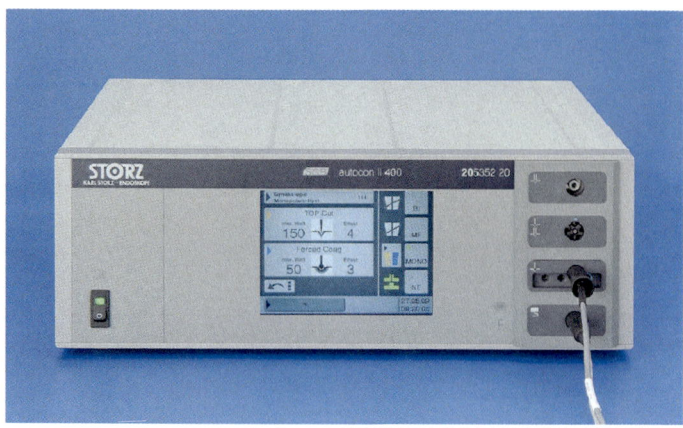

Fig. 3.9: High frequency unit Autocon II 400 (Karl Storz ltd) with pre-selected and saved programme for the **monopolar** resection.

Note: Preselected programmes facilitate the handling.

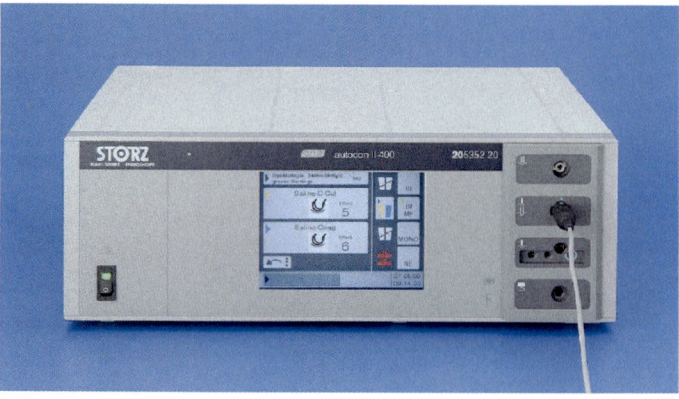

Fig. 3.10: High frequency unit Autocon II 400 (Karl Storz ltd) with pre-selected and saved programme for the **bipolar** resection.

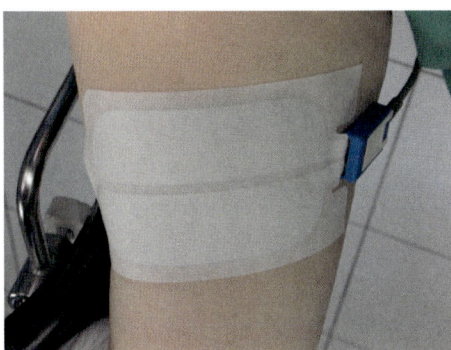

Fig. 3.11: Fixation of the neutral electrode onto the thigh of the patient (only necessary with a monopolar resection).

Note: A correct fixation of the neutral electrode is an important precondition for maximal safety during **monopolar** high frequency surgery.

HF output

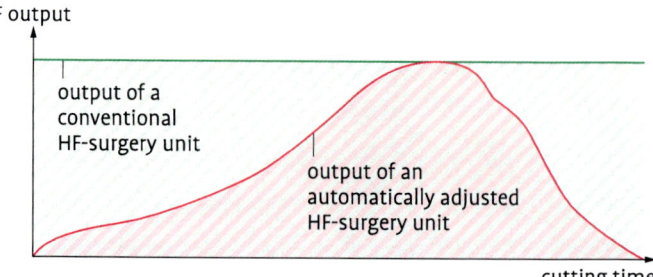

cutting time

Comparison of the output

cutting depth

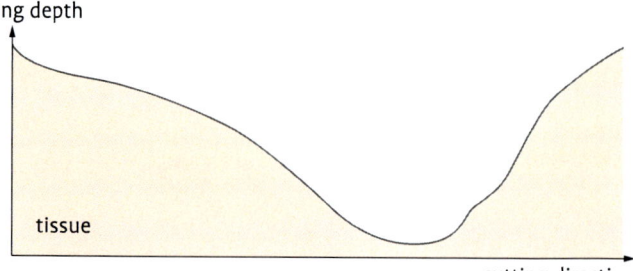

cutting direction

Side view of the cut

Fig. 3.12: Comparison of the necessary output level of an automatically adjusted HF unit and a conventional HF unit.
Upper diagram: The green area shows the output of a conventional HF-surgery unit. The red area shows the output of an automatically adjusted HF-surgery unit.
Lower diagram: Cut from left to right with varying cutting depth. The required power output of an automatically adjusted HF-surgery unit is directly proportional to the cutting depth.

Note: A markedly lower output level when cutting with an automatically adjusted high frequency surgery unit results in a higher safety level.

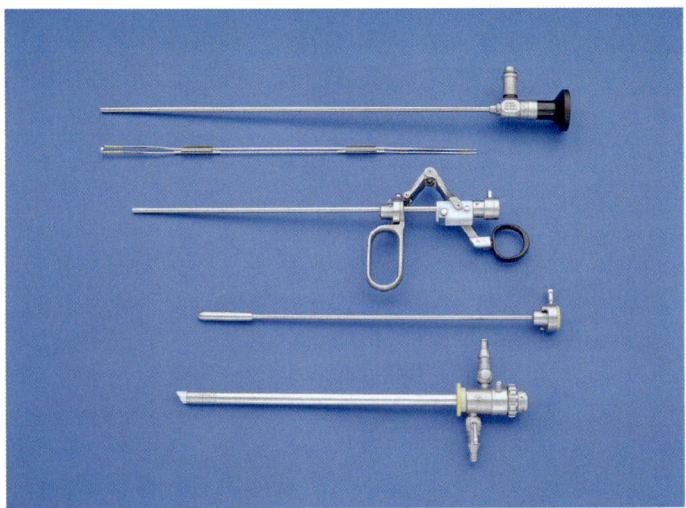

Fig. 3.13: Parts of the hysteroresectoscope for the **bipolar** resection:
- 12° lenses
- electrode
- bipolar resectoscope
- obturator for insertion
- outer and inner sheath with in- and outflow tubes for the distending medium

Note: In contrast to the monopolar roller-ball the bipolar coagulation electrode is fixed and cannot rotate.

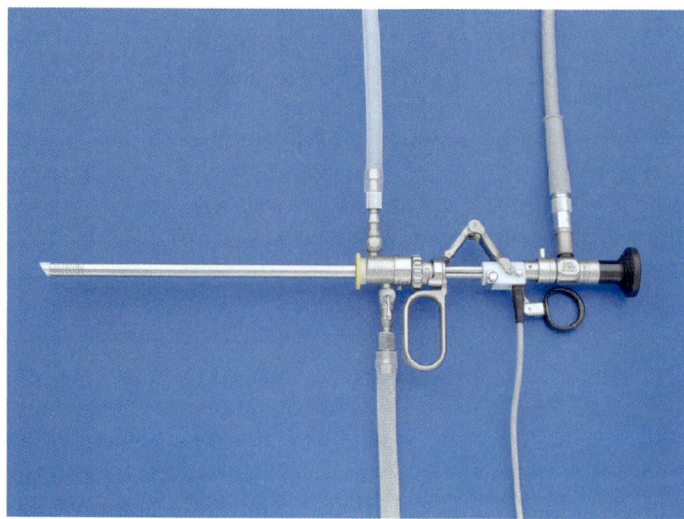

Fig. 3.14: Bipolar hysteroscope (passive element), assembled:
top: supply tube for the distending medium; connection of the light cable
bottom: tube for the outflow of the distending medium; connection of the high frequency unit Autocon II 400

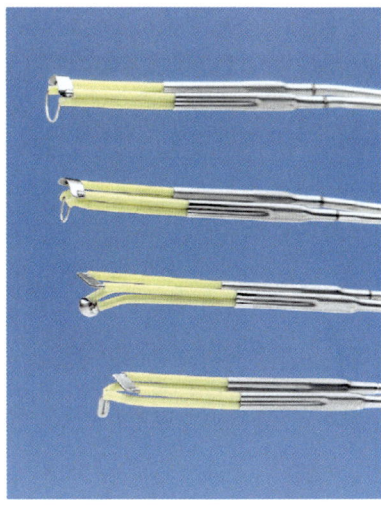

Fig. 3.15: Electrodes for a bipolar resectoscope:
- resection loop (large)
- resection loop (small)
- coagulation electrode
- dissection needle

Distending media

Note: Choose different distending media for a monopolar or a bipolar hysteroscopy.

monopolar	bipolar
electrolyte-free!Sorbitol-Mannitol-solution (Dextran, Glykokol)	**electrolyte-containing!** Ringer's solution (saline solution)

Possible distending media for intrauterine monopolar electrosurgical operations:

Precondition: electrolyte-free solution
- Dextran (Hyskon)
  Disadvantages: possible anaphylactic reactions, possible pulmonary oedemas, encrustation of the lenses

Table 7.1: (Continued)

	uterus bicornis	uterus septus
laparoscopy	fundus uteri: deep median notch	fundus uteri: even or little median raphe
therapy	none; after 3 abortions abdominal or laparo-scopic metroplasty should be considered	hysteroscopic septum dissection

Note: Part of the diagnostics of uterus malformations is the exclusion of renal or ureteral anomalies, which are more frequent among these patients.

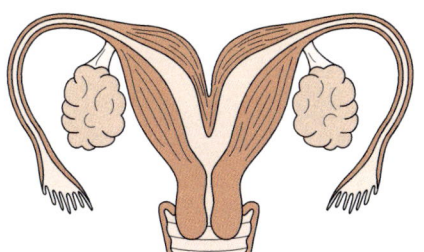

Fig. 7.1:
uterus bicornis; laparo-scopy: deep raphe – bipartite uterus.

Therapy: abdominal or laparoscopic metroplasty with tendency towards habitual abortions

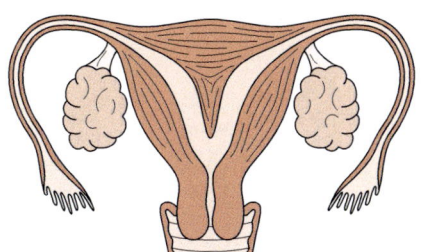

Fig. 7.2:
uterus septus; laparo-scopy: fundus – even or little median raphe.

Therapy: hysteroscopic septum dissection

- Glykokol (Glycin)
  Disadvantages: with overloading possible ammonia intoxication and reversible impaired vision
- Sorbitol-Mannitol-solution
  Disadvantages: no specific disadvantages known

Note: The intrauterine monopolar electrosurgery is only possible with an electrolyte-free fluid distending medium. In Germany we almost exclusively use a Sorbitol-Mannitol-solution.

Note: Never use a saline or Ringer's solution for intrauterine **monopolar** surgery. Risk of burns: cutting process not possible with modern high frequency units! (▶ page 10)

Characteristics of a Sorbitol-Mannitol-solution

1. absolutely abacterial and pyrogen-free
2. sterile
3. clear, makes good view without streaks possible
4. non-conductive
5. not hemolytic
6. inexpensive
7. available in demand-oriented quantities and in user-friendly form (flexible bags of 1.5; 3 and 5 l; canisters of 10 l)
8. sugar alcohol of 3.24%, osmolarity of approximately 180 mosm/l (hypo-osmolar)
9. does not crystallise on the endoscope or the surgical glove
10. quick elimination through metabolisation in the liver (Sorbit) combined with the diuretic effect of Mannit
11. CAVE: fructose intolerance!

Advantages of Ringer's solution:

1. only to be used for **bipolar** electrosurgery
2. no electrolyte shift with fluid overload (higher safety for the patients)
3. slightly more cost-saving

Note: Always use solutions **at body temperature**. Otherwise, especially when larger quantities are used, risk of hypothermia of the patient.

Practical application of a Sorbitol-Mannitol-solution or a Ringer's solution as distending medium

The preoperative planning of the surgery should include the selection of the appropriate quantity of the distending medium.

Recommendations:

- septum dissection: 1,0 l
- endometrial ablation (roller ball): 1.5 l
- myoma resection (myoma <3 cm): 3 l
- endometrium resection (cutting loop): 3 l
- myoma resection (myoma >3 cm or multiple myomas): 5 l
- intrauterine adhesiolysis (depending on grade): 1 to 5 l

Advantages of the correct selection of the quantity of the distending medium:

- shorter time of surgery
- with no need to change bags air bubbles within the system can be reduced (reduced risk of air embolism)
- cost-saving

Note: A fructose intolerance (contraindication for the use of a Sorbitol-Mannitol-solution) is extremely rare. Ask patients about tropical fruits tolerance! On the suspicion of fructose intolerance Glycin should be used as distending medium for the monopolar surgery. However, the bipolar surgery with Ringer's solution as distending medium should be preferred in these cases.

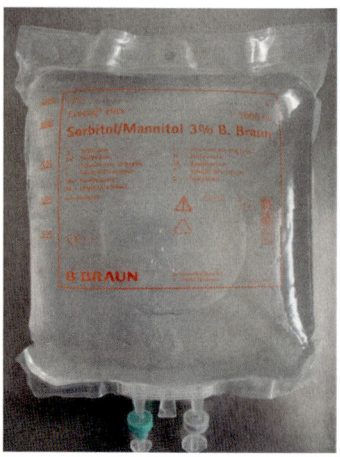
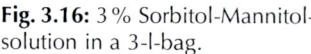

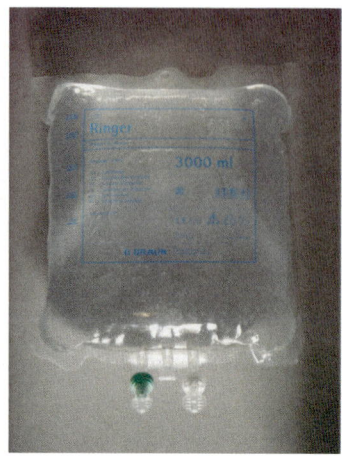

Fig. 3.16: 3 % Sorbitol-Mannitol-solution in a 3-l-bag.

Fig. 3.17: Ringer's solution in a 3-l-bag.

4 Positioning, preparation of surgery and ergonomics

1. positioning of the patient in lithotomy position
2. covering of the surgical area
3. disinfection of the outer genitals and the vagina
4. creation of the best possible conditions for the surgery (ergonomics of surgery!)

From an ergonomic point of view the following conditions should be checked before beginning the surgery:
1. height adjustment of the table
2. monitor in line of view
3. foot pedal within easy reach
4. cable (in- and outflow tube, light and electrical cable) should be within easy reach; if necessary they should be placed on an additional table or be held by a surgical nurse

Note: Placing the cables on a table or having a surgical nurse hold the cables reduces the physical strain for the surgeon especially during longer surgery and prevents the inflow and outflow tubes from bending.

Potential sources of problems during hysteroscopic surgery are:
- table too high (see Fig. 4.1)
- uncomfortable position of the monitor (see Fig. 4.2)
- blinding surgical light (see Fig. 4.3)

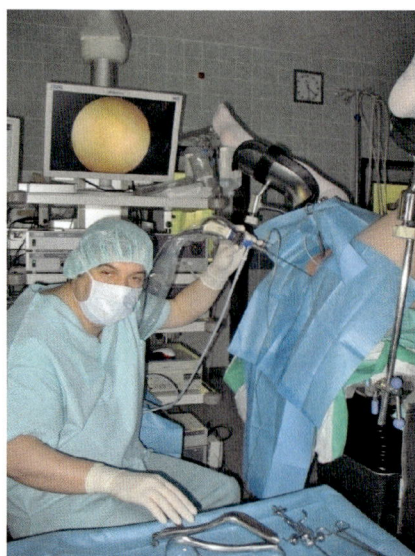

Fig. 4.1:
Table too high.

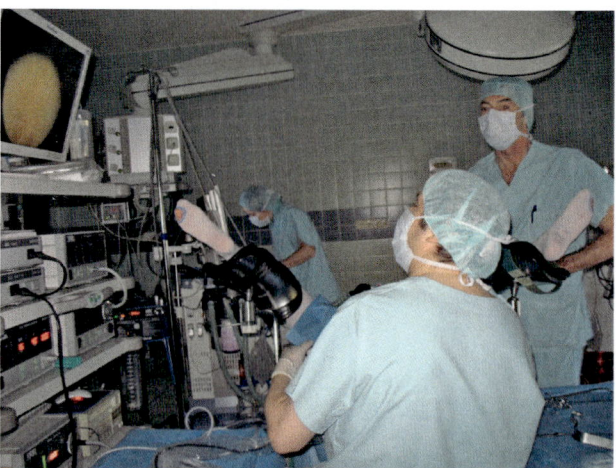

Fig. 4.2: Uncomfortable position of the monitor.

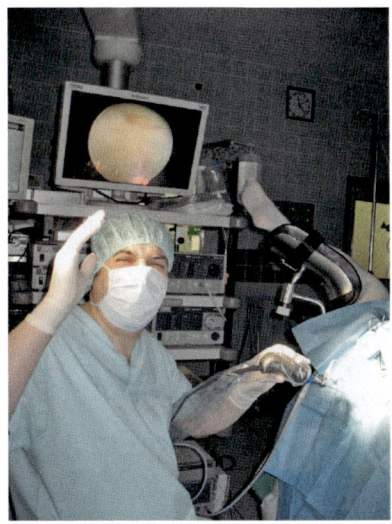

Fig. 4.3:
Blinding surgical light.

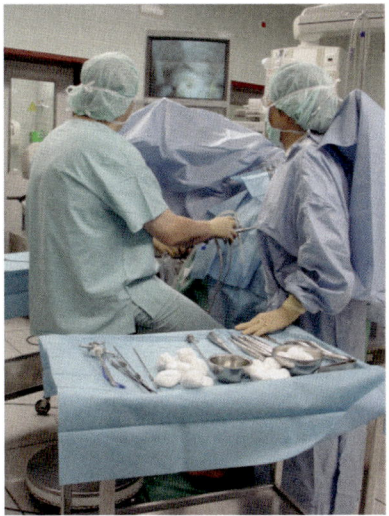

Fig. 4.4:
Ideal conditions for surgery.

5 Technique and procedure of operative hysteroscopy

1. diagnostic hysteroscopy with 5-mm-hysteroscope (procedure described in *Diagnostic Hysteroscopy. Practical Guide*, 2nd edition, deGruyter 2010)
2. dilatation of the cervical canal up to Hegar 9 (when using a smaller resectoscope for fertility surgery up to Hegar 7)
3. insertion of the outer sheath with obturator
4. replacement of the obturator by a hysteroresectoscope with matching electrode and **12° angle lenses**
5. checking of the connections
   a) check of the correct distending medium (bipolar: Ringer's solution; monopolar: Sorbitol-Mannitol-solution)
   b) inflow tube for the distending medium – airless and connected with the hysteromat (irrigate beforehand!)
   c) check of the pressure and flow selection on the hysteromat
   d) outlet tube in collect container
   e) connection with electrosurgical unit and check of the power level on the high frequency unit (preselected programmes for monopolar and bipolar surgery)
6. opening of the inflow tube and distension of the cavum uteri often an irrigation is primarily necessary because the dilatation of the cervix often causes bleedings in the cavum uteri
7. start of the surgery as soon as view and distension are sufficient

Note: Outflow open: good irrigation, bad distension; outflow closed: no irrigation, good distension.

Practical advice: A half-open outflow tap leads to a good distension with sufficient irrigation.

6 Staff requirements

Surgeon

- experience in about 200 diagnostic hysteroscopies performed by him-/herself
- knowledge of indications, contraindications and, first of all, safety aspects of operative hysteroscopy
- knowledge of the fundamentals, safety aspects and complications of electrosurgery
- training with animal models (handling of the equipment)
- knowledge of potential complications and their clinical management
- work shadowing with a surgeon experienced in operative hysteroscopy

Surgical nurse

- exact knowledge of the equipment and instrumentation
- assembly of the hysteroresectoscope
- operation of the hysteromat
- distending medium (selection)
- high frequency unit (adjustments)

Anaesthesiologist

- knowledge of the complications of operative hysteroscopy
- special diagnostics and therapy of the TUR-syndrome or diagnostics and management of air embolism

7 Surgical interventions

7.1 Septum dissection

Indication

Absolute:
- habitual abortions (2 or 3 recurrent abortions)

Relative:
- primary and secondary infertility
- dysmenorrhoea (therapy-resistant)

Note: Subtle preoperative diagnostics is necessary. For a differential diagnosis between uterus bicornis and uterus septus a laparoscopy is imperative.

Note: Never perform a septum dissection without a self-performed or well-documented laparoscopy. **Risk of perforation** with a uterus bicornis!

Table 7.1: Differential diagnosis: uterus bicornis – uterus septus.

	uterus bicornis	uterus septus
incidence	rare uterus malformation	most frequent uterus malformation
rate of abortion without therapy	30%	90%
rate of births at term without therapy	30%	<5%
HSG/hysteroscopy	bipartite cavum	bipartite cavum

Technique of septum dissection

- dissection of the septum with the resection needle from caudal to fundal
- from time to time check of the extent of the dissection using the tubal ostia as points of orientation
- with complete septa first dissect the area caudal, afterwards insert the resectoscope completely (sufficient flow), Fig. 7.3
- then dissection from fundal to caudal, Fig. 7.4
- permanent orientation at the tubal ostia

Note: Dissection in the middle of the septum! Median dissection not up to the ostia level if median raphe is known! **Risk of perforation!** The reconstruction of the cavum uteri as a uterus arcuatus is sufficient for the optimization of fertility.

Note: Spare the tubal ostia when dissection (about 1 cm distance with cutting current) to avoid functional disorders of the ostia.

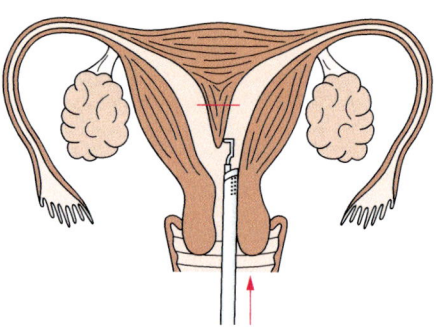

Fig. 7.3: Septum dissection in the caudal area.

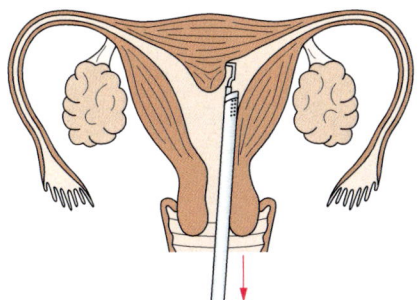

Fig. 7.4: Septum dissection in the fundal area.

Diagnostics and therapeutic management of suspected uterus malformation (uterus septus/bicornis)

1. anamnesis (abortions, premature births?)
2. gynaecological examination and sonography ("two-cavities-phenomenon")
3. scheduling of the surgery – ideally post menstruationem (thin endometrium)
4. procedure of the surgery:
   diagnostic hysteroscopy: cavum uteri divided into two parts
   b) diagnostic laparoscopy: fundus of the uterus smooth or small median raphe
   diagnosis: uterus septus
   c) when indicated, simultaneous laparoscopic resection of the endometriosis
   d) operative hysteroscopy with transcervical septum dissection (with complete septa perhaps insertion of an IUD to prevent adhesions)

Note: A treatment with GnRH-analogues before the septum dissection does not bring any intra- or postoperative advantages and can therefore be waived if surgery is performed post menstruationem.

Reference:

Römer T: The value of GnRH agonist treatments before hysteroscopic septum dissection. Zentralbl. Gynakl 1998; 120: 42–4

Case report of a 29-year-old patient

1. Clinical diagnosis: uterus septus
2. Anamnesis: sonographically suspected uterus malformation with dysmenorrhoea and desire to have children
3. Sonography: 2 endometrial islands
4. Hysteroscopy: septum reaching to the inner cervix (4.5 cm)
5. Therapy: laparoscopy: fundus of the uterus smooth and wide, resection of the endometriosis, transcervical septum dissection and insertion of an IUD

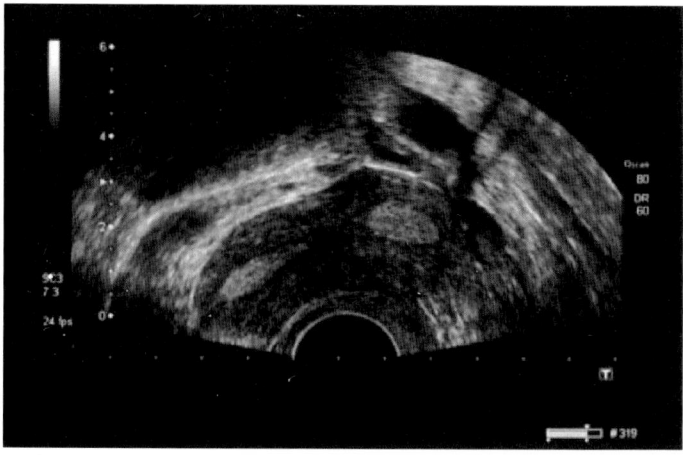

Fig. 7.5: Vaginal sonography: in the cross section 2 endometrial islands ("two-cavities-phenomenon").

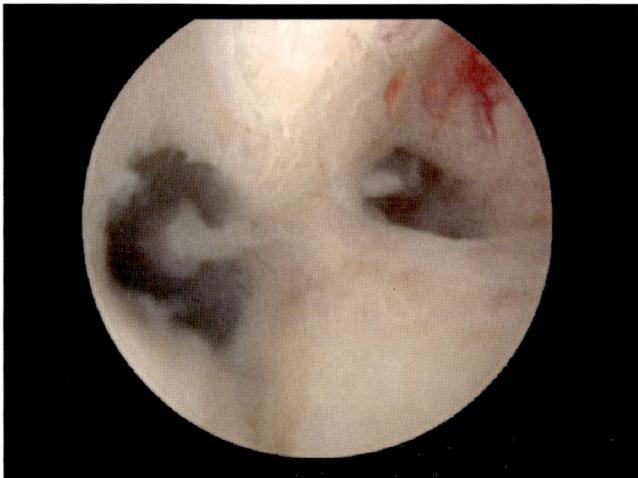

Fig. 7.6: Diagnostic hysteroscopy: uterus septus/bicornis.

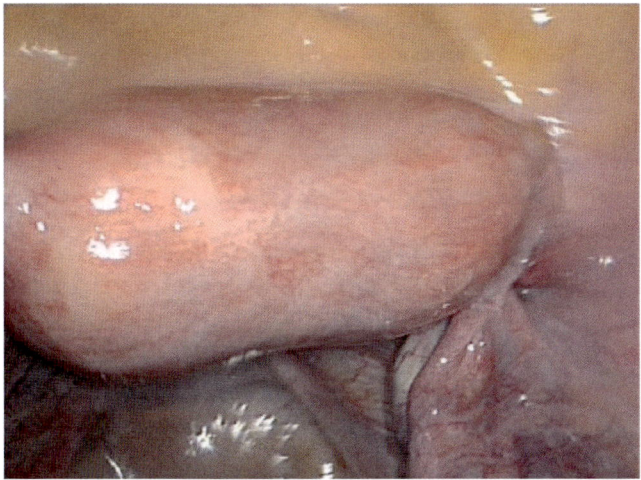

Fig. 7.7: Diagnostic laparoscopy: uterus wide and smooth.

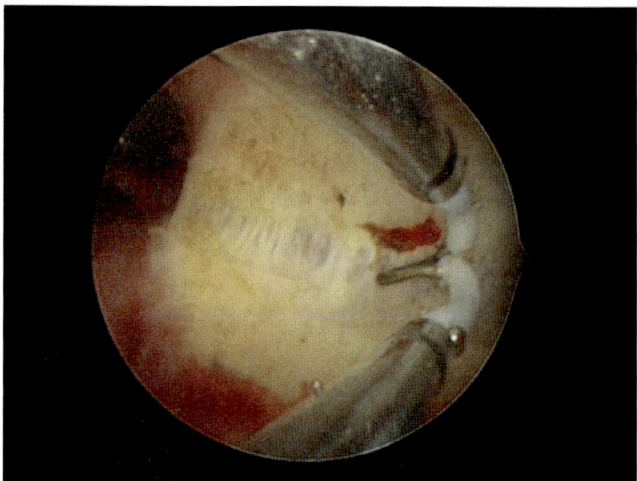

Fig. 7.8: Transcervical septum dissection.

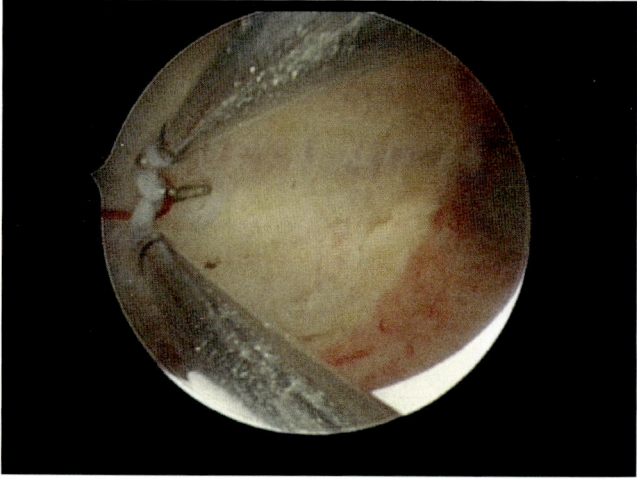

Fig. 7.9: Final findings of a normal cavum uteri after septum dissection.

Procedure of a septum dissection

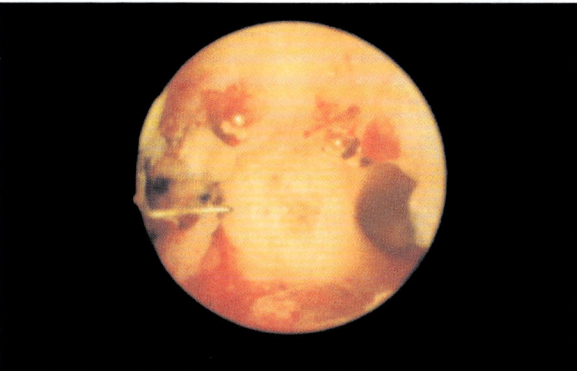

Fig. 7.10: Septum dissection in a patient suffering from habitual abortions – beginning of surgery.

- typical cords from anterior to posterior wall by distension permanent stretching of the septum cords at first dissection from caudal to fundal until sufficient intracavitary space and view to change the direction of the dissection are gained

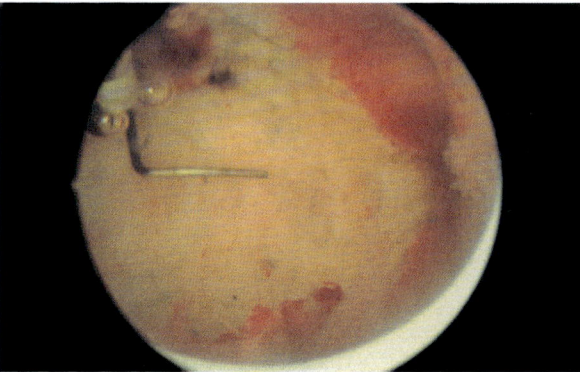

Fig. 7.11: Septum dissection: septum has already been removed caudally. Now further orientation towards the tubal ostia and further dissection from lateral to medial and from fundal to caudal.

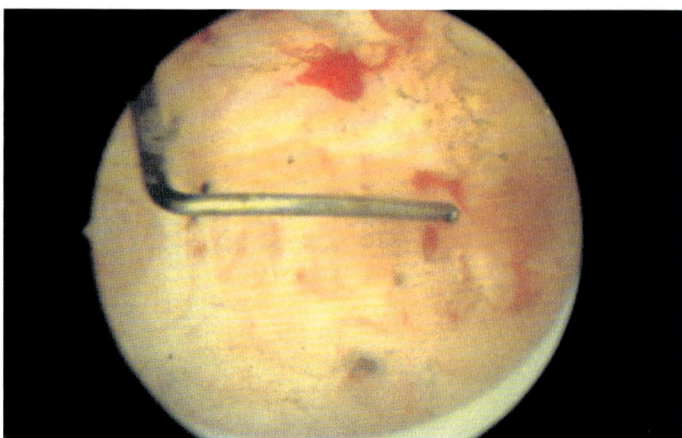

Fig. 7.12: Septum dissection in a patient suffering from habitual abortions – end of surgery; beginning bleeding from single myometrial vessels.
→ stop surgery, otherwise very high risk of perforation!

Note: The use of a thin hysteroresectoscope (outer diameter 7 mm) is of advantage with a septum dissection (better distension and irrigation in a narrow cavity)

Uterus septus completus

- very rare special form of a uterus septus
- often associated with a vaginal septum
- complete cervical and corporal septum
- subtle prediagnostics necessary

Differential diagnosis:
- uterus bicornis bicollis
- uterus didelphys (duplex)

Question: Dissection of the cervical septum?

Practical advice: Dissection of the corporal septum with preservation of the cervical septum to prevent premature births.

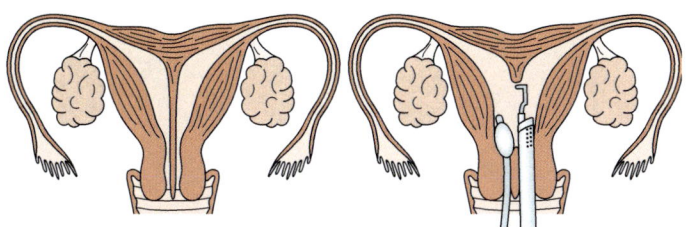

Fig. 7.13: Dissection of the corporal septum with preservation of the cervical septum of a uterus septus completes by means of Balloon-technique.

Advantages of the Balloon-technique:
1. Orientation for the „blind" perforation of the corporal septum
2. Prevention of losing distending medium through the second cervical canal during septum dissection

Reference:

Römer T, Lober R: Hysteroscopic correction of a complete septate uterus using a balloon technique. Hum Reprod 1997; 12: 478–9

Septum dissection after abdominal metroplasty

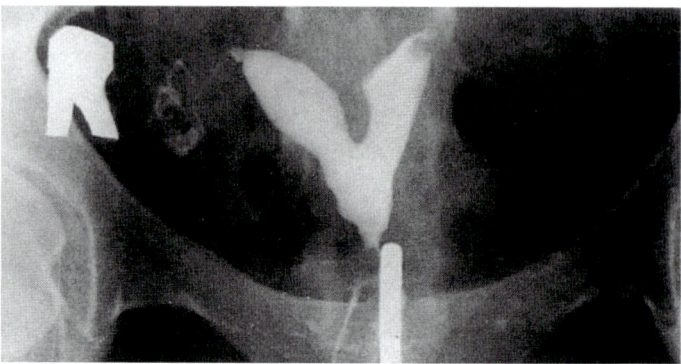

Fig. 7.14: HSG-findings after abdominal metroplasty with residual septum.

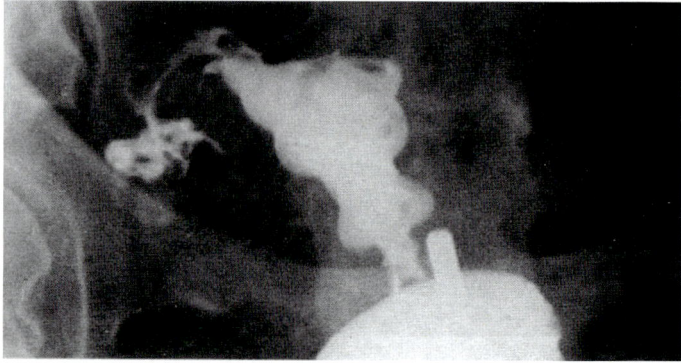

Fig. 7.15: HSG-findings of the same patient after hysteroscopic dissection of the residual septum.

Note: Even residual septum after primary abdominal metroplasty can be hysteroscopically dissected. No relaparotomy necessary!

Postoperative management after septum dissection

With complete or wide septa or additional intrauterine adhesions
- at the end of the surgery insertion of an IUD for the prevention of intrauterine adhesions for the duration of 3 months (preferably IUD type DANA or copper-IUD with a wide surface)
- oestrogenisation for 3 months to stimulate the endometrium proliferation (e.g. 2–4 mg oestradiol for 21 days progestagen for 12 days)
- follow-up hysteroscopy (possibly with IUD extraction), in most of the cases as outpatient procedure without anaesthesia, possible after 3 months

Note: An IUD-insertion und oestrogenisation is only recommended with complete septa for the prevention of possible adhesions (lack of sufficient data).

Frequent combination of uterus malformation and endometriosis (up to 50 %)

Cave: No oestrogenisation with evidence of an endometriosis.

Note: With simultaneous occurrence of a uterus septus and an endometriosis the endometriosis should be removed as completely as possible by a laparoscopy (preoperative information of the patient!).

Note: A treatment with GnRH-analogues after septum dissection and endometrium resection is **not** recommended because after a septum dissection an endometrium proliferation is of greater advantage for the healing of the wound.

**Most frequent complications of the septum dissection:
Perforation in the fundal area**

Management:
- diagnostic laparoscopy
- check for injuries of other organs (especially bowel injuries); if these cannot be definitely excluded, a laparotomy is indicated!
- with bleeding – endoscopic suture for haemostasis
- perioperative application of antibiotics
- frequent post-operative follow-up

Cave: After uterus perforation during the septum dissection there is an increased risk of a uterus rupture with later pregnancies (28th to 34th week of pregnancy!). Close prepartal supervision and generous indication for a caesarean section! Preoperative information of the patient about this potential complication is necessary!

Prevention of the perforation of the fundus during a hysteroscopic septum dissection

- consideration of the median raphe (median dissection in the fundal area not as far as in the lateral area)
- with beginning bleeding from the vessels in the septum area – stop surgery because these are mainly myometrial vessels (during a teaching surgery possibly septum dissection under simultaneous sonographic or laparoscopic control)
- with indistinct orientation about the level of the dissection – simultaneous abdominal sonography
- in most of the cases laparoscopy is only useful after perforation!

Note: In infertile patients the operative hysteroscopy should only be performed by a surgeon experienced in hysteroscopy!

Table 7.2: Comparison of abdominal metroplasty and transcervical septum dissection.

	Abdominal metroplasty	Hysteroscopic septum dissection
Approach	laparotomy	transcervical
Average duration of surgery	120 min	15 min
Possible secondary complications caused by surgery	intraperitoneal adhesions	perforation
postoperative birth-rate	80–90 %	80–90 %
Opening of the uterine cavity	yes	no
obstetric management	higher frequency of Caesarean ections (no primary indication for a caesarean section)	no indication for a Caesarean section

Note: Today the hysteroscopic septum dissection is the standard therapy for the uterus septus. There is no indication for an abdominal metroplasty with a uterus septus!

Success rates of the hysteroscopic septum dissection

Table 7.3: Meta analysis (literature) of the success rates of the hystero-scopic septum dissection 709 patients (1986–2000).

	preoperative	postoperative
abortion rate	77.4–88.9%	8.2–27.7%
live-birth-rate	8.9–22.6%	59.6–91.8%

Table 7.4: Own results with hysteroscopic septum dissection Patients suffering from habitual abortions and secondary infertility 123 patients (1995–2005) with follow-up (24–60 months).

	preoperative	postoperative
abortion rate	68.5%	11.9%
live-birth-rate	17.7%	78.6%

7.2 Intrauterine adhesiolysis

Indication

- habitual abortions (2 or more recurrent abortions)
- primary and secondary infertility
- hypomenorrhea/amenorrhea
- dysmenorrhea
- recurrent lower abdominal pain

Note: Strict indication for intrauterine adhesiolysis for grades III and IV because this is the most difficult operative-hysteroscopic intervention with a high rate of complications.

Table 7.5: Intrauterine adhesions – classification according to the European Society of Hysteroscopy (ESGE).

grade I	thin, filmy adhesions • can be easily cut with the sheath of the hysteroscope • cornual areas normal
grade II	singular firm adhesions • in different areas of the cavity • connect uterine walls, but tubal ostia are visible • cannot be cut with sheath of the hysteroscope
grade II A	occluding adhesions only in the internal cervical os, upper uterine cavity normal
grade III	multiple firm adhesions • in different areas • unilateral occlusion of the cornual area
grade III A	extensive scarring of the uterine cavity with amenorrhea or distinctive hypomenorrhea
grade III B	combination of III and III A
grade IV	extensive firm adhesions with agglutination of the anterior and posterior uterine wall and occlusion of both cornual areas

Note: A classification according to the grades is primarily necessary because of its therapeutic and prognostic consequences.

Table 7.6: Operative therapy and prognosis of intrauterine adhesions.

	grade I	grade II	grade III and IV
operative therapy	cutting by sheath of the hysteroscope	cutting by microscissors	electrosurgical adhesiolysis or by laser (operative hysteroscopy)
successful therapy of the bleeding disorders	100%	100%	60–70%
pregnancy rate	70–90%	70–90%	20–40%

Diagnostics and therapeutic management in the case of suspected intrauterine adhesions

1. anamnesis:
   a) bleeding characteristics?
   b) intrauterine intervention!!
2. gynaecological examination
3. vaginal sonography:
   a) endometrium structure
4. diagnostic hysteroscopy:
   a) intrauterine adhesions with description of the grade
5. operative hysteroscopy simultaneous (preoperative information!) with intrauterine adhesiolysis (if necessary, simultaneous sonography or laparoscopy)
6. IUD-insertion at the end of surgery (compulsory with grades III and IV according to ESGE)
7. oestrogenisation for 3 months for endometrium proliferation
8. follow-up hysteroscopy with IUD-extraction (if necessary, further adhesiolysis)

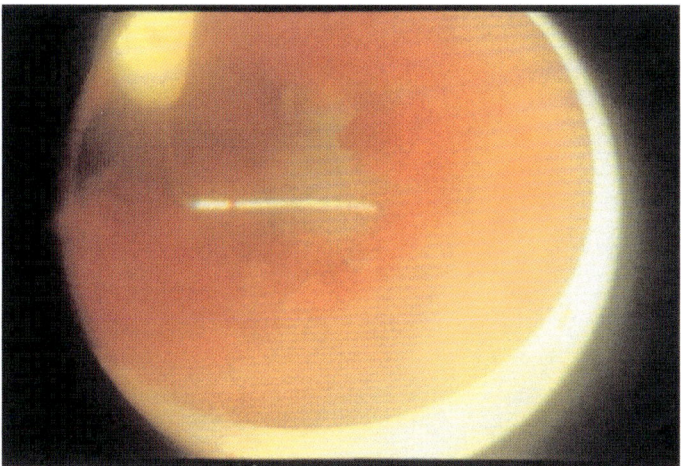

Fig. 7.16: Intrauterine adhesion grade III in a patient suffering from secondary amenorrhea after abortion curettage. One tubal ostium is covered by the adhesive cord.
→ start of the electrosurgical adhesiolysis with the resection needle.

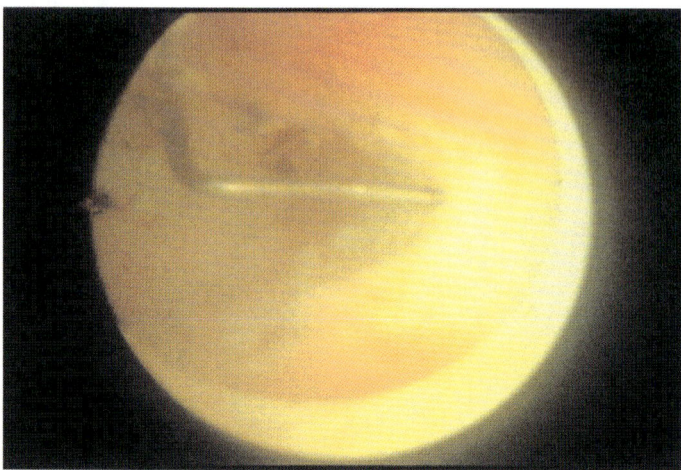

Fig. 7.17: Intrauterine adhesion grade III in the same patient – left tubal ostium exposed.

Note: Careful electrosurgical dissection of adhesions of grades III and IV because of high risk of perforation. Strict indication and extensive preoperative information of the patient necessary!

Case report of a 29-year-old patient

1.	Clinical diagnosis:	intrauterine adhesions grade III
2.	Anamnesis:	3 years ago hysteroscopic myoma resection performed externally, now planned IVF because of tubal and andrological sterility, hypomenorrhea
3.	Sonography:	endometrium only fragmentarily visible
4.	Hysteroscopy:	complete left half of the cavity covered by adhesive cords, right ostium visible (intrauterine adhesions grade III)
5.	Therapy:	operative hysteroscopy, intrauterine electrosurgical adhesiolysis and IUD-insertion

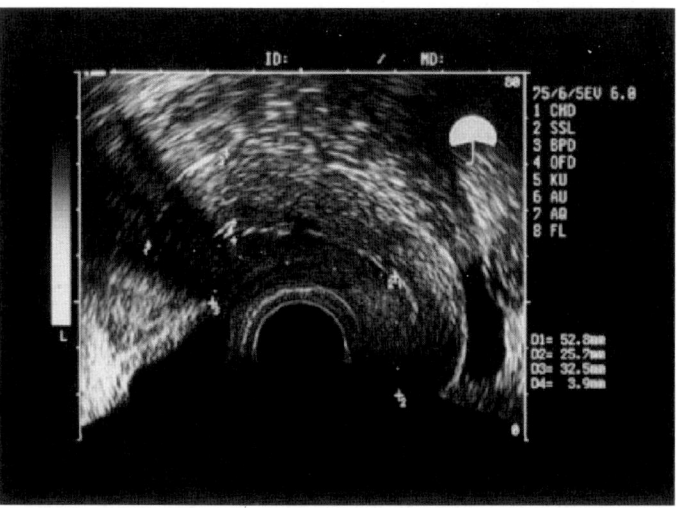

Fig. 7.18: Sonography: endometrium defects, endometrium only fragmentarily visible.

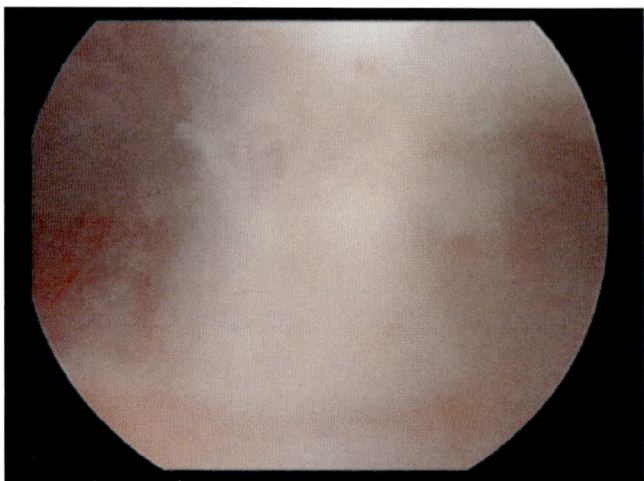

Fig. 7.19: Intrauterine adhesions grade III left half of the cavity.

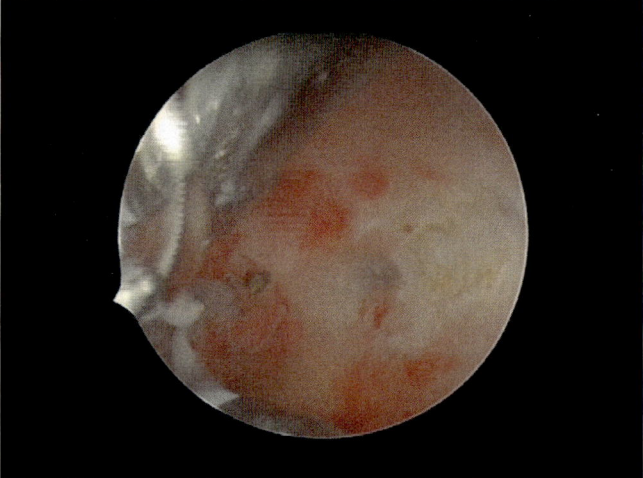

Fig. 7.20: Intrauterine adhesiolysis with exposure of the left ostium.

Case report of a 37-year-old patient

1. Clinical diagnosis: secondary amenorrhea with intrauterine adhesions
2. Anamnesis: 3 years ago postoperative curettage because of residual placenta, afterwards secondary amenorrhea, hormonal status: regular
3. Sonography: endometrium only fragmentarily visible
4. Hysteroscopy: median solid adhesive cord (IUA grade III)
5. Therapy: intrauterine adhesiolysis, IUD-insertion and oestrogenisation

Note: If tubal ostia are not visible, a simultaneous abdominal sonography or laparoscopy is necessary for a better intracavitary orientation.

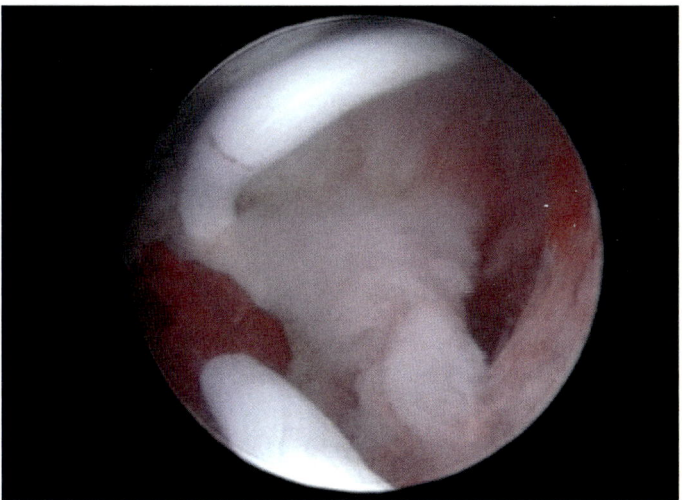

Fig. 7.21: Intrauterine adhesiolysis of the median adhesive cord.

Postoperative management after intrauterine electrosurgical adhesiolysis

compulsory
- insertion of an IUD for 3 months
- oestrogenisation for 3 months
- outpatient follow-up hysteroscopy and IUD-extraction (if necessary, further adhesiolysis) 3 months after surgery

Note: The low postoperative pregnancy and birth rate and the difficult and complicated surgery require focusing one's attention on the prevention of intrauterine adhesions.

Possible prevention of intrauterine adhesions

- strict indication for intrauterine interventions in patients at a fertile age and post partum as well as in childbed
- atraumatic curettages in patients at a fertile age
- generous perioperative application of antibiotics
- post-abortion – hysteroscopy (8 weeks after abortion curettage) with the opportunity of the early diagnostics and therapy of small adhesions
- in infertile patients, myoma resection with care for the endometrium
- careful examination of the placenta post partum (prevention of curettages during childbed – lower danger of adhesions with immediate post-partal curettages compared with curettages during childbed)

Intrauterine electrosurgical adhesiolysis for adhesions of grades III and IV

- high risk of perforation because orientation in the cavity is difficult (tubal ostia as points of orientation are mostly hidden behind adhesive cords)
- most difficult operative hysteroscopy (should only be performed in endoscopic centres)

- successful therapy of menstrual disorders (60-80% of patients: regular menstruation after surgery)
- limited postoperative pregnancy and birth rate (less than 30%)
- subsequent pregnancies and births with a high rate of complications (intrauterine retardations, placenta accreta and increta)

Practical advice: Because of the high risk of perforation a simultaneous sonography or laparoscopy during the dissection of intrauterine adhesions of grades III and IV is recommended.

Anamnesis and results of 48 intrauterine adhesiolyses of grades III and IV/ESGE

Academic Hospital Cologne-Weyertal, 2001–2008

Table 7.7: Causes of intrauterine adhesions of grades III and IV/ESGE (anamnesis!).

Anamnesis	n	%
abortion curettage	19	39.6
post-partal curettage	22	45.8
hysteroscopic myoma resection	6	12.5
laparoscopic myoma enucleation	1	2.1
	48	100.0

Table 7.8: Pre- and postoperative bleeding disorders in patients suffering from intrauterine adhesions grades III and IV/ESGE.

Bleeding patterns	Preoperative [n]	Postoperative [n]
amenorrhea	19	1
hypomenorrhea	24	11
eumenorrhea	5	36
	48	48

Table 7.9: Postoperative pregnancies after intrauterine adhesiolysis.

48 patients	%	
17 pregnancies	35.4	
12 live births	25.2	
4 abortions	8.1	
1 EUP	2.1	

Pseudo-Asherman-syndrome

- false diagnosis of intrauterine adhesions grade IV with via falsa into the myometrium (e.g. with a cervical stenosis)

Note: If there is no anamnestic correlation to intrauterine interventions and associated changes of the bleeding patterns, intrauterine adhesions grade IV can almost always be excluded (exception: genital tuberculosis).

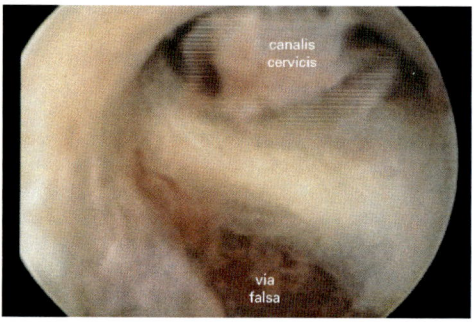

Fig. 7.22: Pseudo-Asherman-syndrome.
Referral of the patient with the diagnosis of a Pseudo-Asherman-syndrome.
Hysteroscopy: via falsa on the posterior wall of the cervix.

Reference:

Römer T; Lober R: Asherman's Syndrome as a Frequent Wrong Diagnosis of a 'Via Falsa' in Hysteroscopic Diagnosis of Sterile Patients. Geburtsh Frauenheilk 1998; 58: 328–30

7.3 Myoma resection

Indications for hysteroscopic myoma resection

- recurrent bleeding disorders resistant to therapy, in most of the cases connected with dysmenorrhoea or secondary anaemia
- bleeding disorders during oral contraception or postmenopausal hormone therapy
- habitual abortions
- primary and secondary infertility

Note: A hysteroscopic resection is only indicated for solitary submucous myomas! In patients with multiple intramural myomas the resection of a solitary submucous myoma is no alternative to the hysterectomy or just a temporary solution (high rate of failure).

Exception: Multiple myomas without any further discomfort in perimenopausal patients suffering from bleeding disorders caused by a submucous myoma

Submucous myomas and infertility

Note: Submucous myomas can cause implantation problems and thus reduce the pregnancy rate. Large submucous myomas cause a rise in the frequency of abortions.

Table 7.10: Influence of myomas on fertility.

Position of the myoma	Influence
submucous	+++
intramural	+
subserous	∅

Note: The closer the myoma is located at the endometrium, the higher is the probability of fertility disorders.

Fertility and hysteroscopic myomas resection

Table 7.11: Influence of submucous myomas on the abortion rate.

	Hysteroscopic myoma resection	
	before	after
Live birth rate	3.8 %	63.2 %
Abortion rate	61.6 %	26.3 %

Reference:

Shokeir TA: Hysteroscopic management in submucous fibroids to improve fertility. Arch Gynecol Obstet 2005; 273: 50–4

Classification of submucous myomas

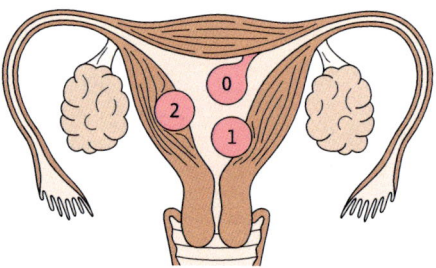

Fig. 7.23: Groups of myomas based on the ESGE classification: Grade 0: no intramural portion; grade 1: intramural portion <50 %; grade 2: intramural portion >50 %.

Note: Only myomas of grades 0 and 1 are suited for a routine hysteroscopic myoma resection.

With a grade-2-myoma the benefit-risk-ratio has to be especially carefully assessed.

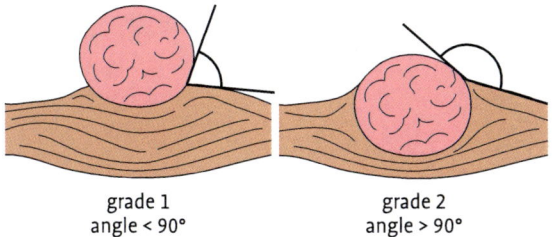

grade 1
angle < 90°

grade 2
angle > 90°

Fig. 7.24: Differentiation between grade-1- and grade-2-myomas based on the angular degree.

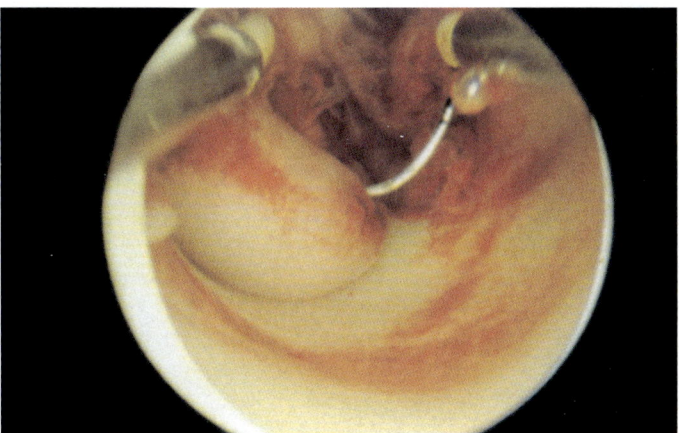

Fig. 7.25: Submucous myoma grade 0/ESGE (complete myoma situated in the cavity – easy resection possible).

Note: Gradual resection of the myoma. Cutting of the peduncle is possible but the transcervical removal in toto is not possible without extended cervical dilatation.

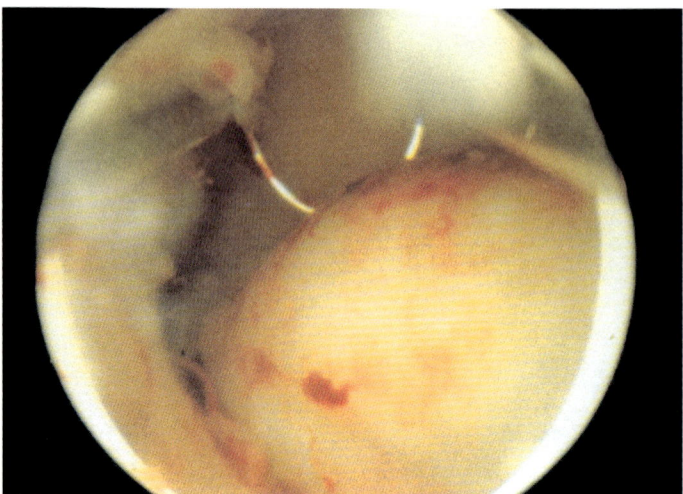

Fig. 7.26: Submucous myoma grade 1/ESGE (intramural portion <50 %).
- resection possible without problems
- intramural portion is pressed towards the cavity by the contraction of the uterus

Note: The intramural portion has to be resected with special care. Small resectates to be preferred. Myoma capsule easily palpable with the cutting loop (outer edge of myoma).

Note: By the intraoperative administration of Methergin® (i.v. injection) the uterus contracts and the intramural portion is pressed into the cavity.

Practical application

Inject 1 ampoule Methergin-injection solution slowly i.v. (0.2 mg Methylergometrine).

The administration of Methergin® for this indication is off-label use and is contraindicated for patients with coronary pre-existing conditions.

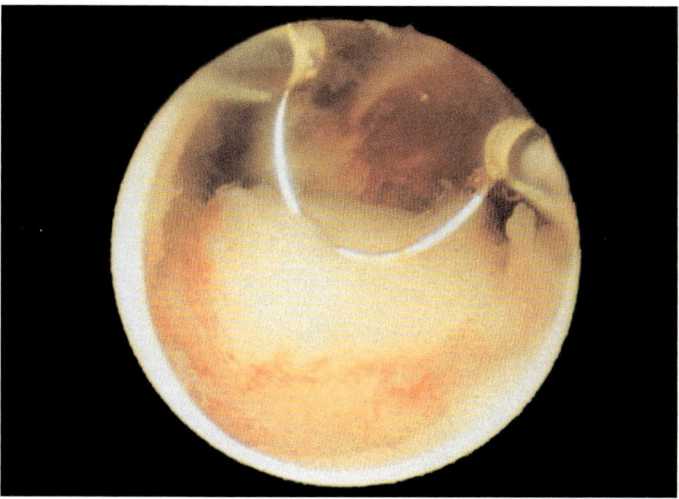

Fig. 7.27: Submucous myoma grade 2/ESGE, intramural portion >50%-high risk of perforation!

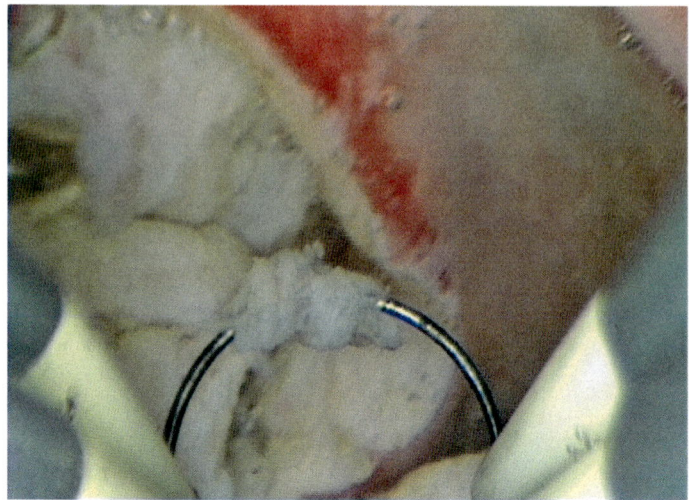

Fig. 7.28: Bipolar myoma resection of a submucous myoma grade 2.

Intramural myomas grade 2 (ESGE)

- strict indication for any surgical treatment of myomas grade 2 (ESGE)
- sonographic safety distance serosa – myoma capsule should be 5 (better even 8) mm
- high risk of perforation (with risk of bowel injury)
- surgery should be performed by a surgeon experienced in operative hysteroscopy

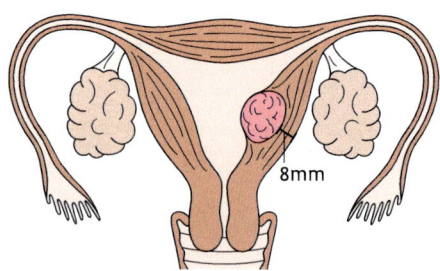

Fig. 7.29: Intramural myoma (grade 2/ ESGE), safety distance between myoma capsule and serosa: 8 mm.

Note: Efficient preoperative sonographic diagnostics increases intraoperative safety.

Special features of myomas grade 2 (ESGE)

Note: After the resection of the submucous myoma portion the intramural portion often bulges out into the uterine cavity by uterus contraction, and can then be resected. This can be stimulated by the i.v. administration of methylergometrine (Methergin®). (▶ page 52)

Note: With a difficult intraoperative view of the cavity (by bleedings or floating myoma resectates) it is better to perform a second-session-surgery. The patient should already be informed of this option in advance.

When using the bipolar technique this risk of multiple surgeries is considerably reduced. (▶ page 105).

Note: The safety of a myoma resection is increased by a simultaneous intraoperative abdominal sonography. A laparoscopy is in most of the cases only useful after a perforation!

Note: The perforation of the uterus by the cutting loop without a definite exclusion of a thermal lesion of adjacent organs (bowels, bladder) justifies a laparotomy (preoperative information)!

For the preoperative information special information forms should be used (e.g. perimed Compliance Verlag, Erlangen).

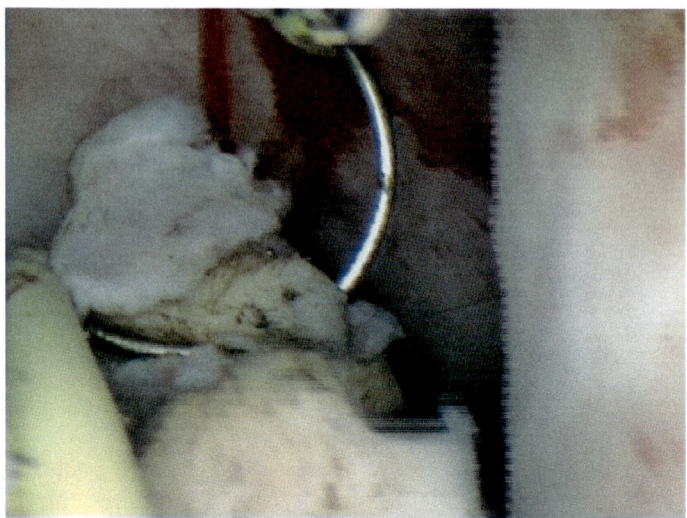

Fig. 7.30: Multiple submucous myomas (about 10) in an infertile patient, bipolar myoma resection in 2 sessions.

Note: With multiple submucous myomas and in infertile patients the limits of hysteroscopic surgery are reached. In these cases the only therapeutic option is hysteroscopic surgery, if necessary in several sessions.

Indications for the bipolar myoma resection

compulsory
- myoma resection of multiple myomas with expected longer duration of surgery
- intrauterine myomas (grade 2/ESGE) with anticipated higher fluid volume deficit during surgery

optional
- myoma resection in patients suffering from infertility (more gentle to the endometrium?)

Note: For a myoma resection the primary use of the bipolar technique should always be considered. (▶ p. 103)

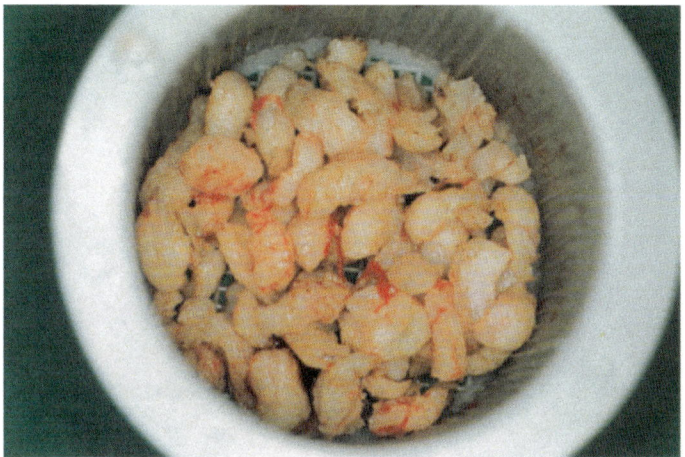

Fig. 7.31: Collecting container in the TUR-apron to collect myoma resectates.

Note: A histological examination of all resectates is absolutely necessary to exclude sarcomas and proliferative leiomyomas. (▶ case report page 127)

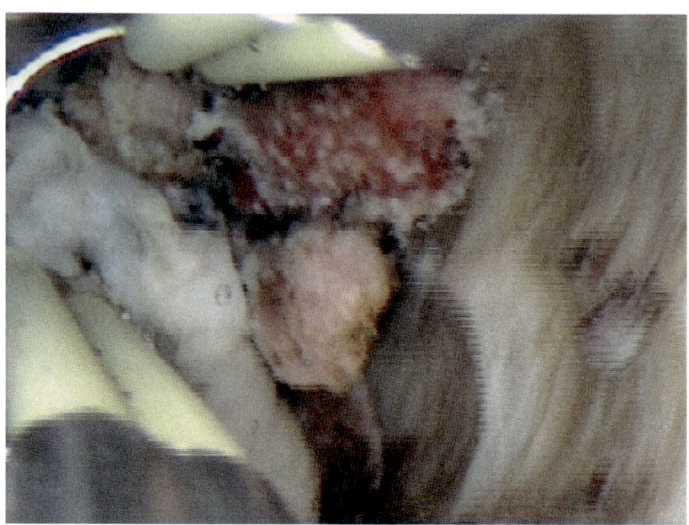

Fig. 7.32: Myoma resection in a patient suffering from menorrhagia; floating resectates obstruct intraoperative view → irrigation and removal of resectates or else high risk of perforation.

Three ways to remove the resectates:
- by blunt curette
- by resectoscope with lying sheath (to be preferred in infertile patients)
- by vacuum suction

Note: In practice the removal of the resectates by a blunt curette has proven effective.

An **alternative** is the so-called Master-resectoscope®, which permits the suction of the resectates.

Disadvantages of the Master-resectoscope®:
- only monopolar technique possible
- additional equipment necessary (suction pump)

Hysteroscopic myoma resection

Time of surgery:
1. without pretreatment: post menstruationem (best: first or second day without bleeding)
2. with pretreatment with GnRH- analogues: 2–3 weeks after last injection

Indications for the use of GnRH-analogues before the hysteroscopic myoma resection:
1. in all infertile patients with submucous myomas of a diameter >3 cm
2. with unfavourable position of the myoma (e.g. in the tubal corner)
3. with secondary anaemia caused by bleeding disorders (auto-reinfusion)
4. with larger intramural myomas (grade 2/ESGE)
5. with myomas that cannot be completely resected during one session

Aim of the application of GnRH-analogues:
- reduction of the myoma volume
- suppression of the endometrium
- with secondary anaemia: normalisation of the Hb-parameter by the induced amenorrhea

Advantages of the pretreatment with GnRH-analogues

- shorter duration of surgery
- better intraoperative view because of less bleedings
- low intraoperative blood loss
- low fluid deficit (lower probability of overloading)
- less complications (reduced risk of perforation especially with unfavourably located myomas)
- desired postoperative effect
- higher compliance than oral medication – simple method of application (one injection – 4-weeks-effect)

- surgery can be flexibly scheduled (independent of menstruation)
- higher preoperative Hb-data (adjustment of secondary anaemia)
- no menstruation when multi-session surgeries are necessary

Disadvantages of the application of GnRH-analogues before hysteroscopic myoma resections

- costs
- side effects (however, in most of the cases only relevant after 3rd injection)
- sometimes more difficult dilatation of the cervical canal
- sometimes myomas are too soft (lack of resistance during resection)

Pretreatment with GnRH-analogues

Beginning of treatment: variable
When beginning in the second half of the menstrual cycle – prior exclusion of pregnancy necessary!
Duration of treatment: at least 2 injections at intervals of 4 weeks (sometimes a 3rd injection may be necessary)

Note: An application of more than 3 injections of GnRH-analogues is only useful in exceptional cases because no further substantial reduction in volume of the myoma can be expected. Apart from that, the side effects as well as the costs increase.

Note: Before a pretreatment with GnRH-analogues are careful benefit-risk-analysis is necessary. A pretreatment with GnRH-analogues is **not compulsory** before a hysteroscopic myoma resection!

Table 7.12: Recommendations for the pretreatment with GnRH-analogues before myoma resections.

Localisation	Diameter of the myoma		
	<3cm	3–6 cm	>6cm
grade 0	–	+	++
grade 1	–	++	+++
grade 2	++	++	+++

–, no indication for pretreatment; +, pretreatment may be considered; ++, indication for pretreatment given; +++, pretreatment absolutely necessary

Results of the hysteroscopic myoma resection with bleeding disorders

Table 7.13: Results of hysteroscopic myoma resections Academic Hospital Cologne-Weyertal, bleeding disorders follow-up 12–36 months.

Localisation	Surgeries	Reduction of bleeding disorders	
	n	n	%
grade 0	64	53	82.8
grade 1	53	41	77.4
grade 2	42	25	59.5
	159	119	74.8

Table 7.14: Results of hysteroscopic myoma resection Academic Hospital Cologne-Weyertal, bleeding disorders follow-up 12–36 months.

	Surgeries	No improvement		Hysterectomy	
	n	n	%	n	%
grade 0	64	11	17.2	2	3.1
grade 1	53	12	22.6	5	9.4
grade 2	42	17	40.5	9	21.4
	159	40	25.2	16	10.1

7.4 Polyp resection

Note: A differentiation between a submucous myoma and a fibrotic corpus polyp by hysteroscopy is not always possible with certainty.

With corpus polyps that cannot be removed mechanically (by target curettage) an operative hysteroscopy with transcervical resection of the polyp may become necessary (preoperative information of the patient is required).

Diagnostic and therapeutic management of corpus polyps

1. gynaecological examination and vaginal sonography, if necessary progesterone test to differentiate between polyp and endometrium hyperplasia)
2. diagnostic hysteroscopy and target curettage
3. follow-up hysteroscopy
4. polyp cannot be removed
5. operative hysteroscopy (patient should already be informed before surgery) with transcervical electrosurgical resection of the polyp

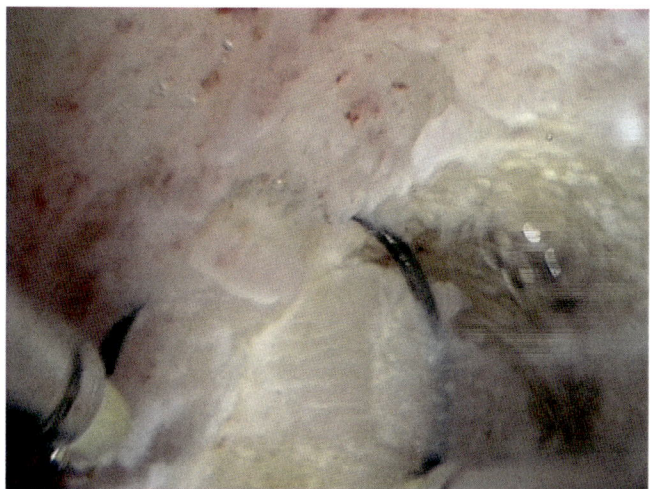

Fig. 7.33: Hysteroscopic polyp resection.

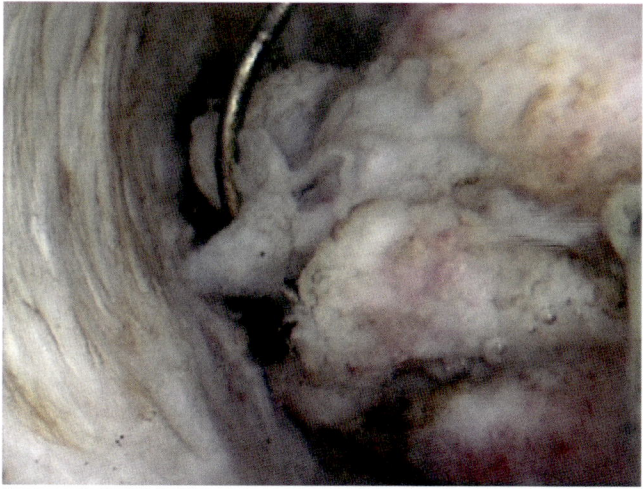

Fig. 7.34: Hysteroscopic polyp resection.

7.5 Endometrial ablation/-resection

Therapeutic possibilities for patients with therapy-resistant recurrent hypermenorrheas without pathological genital findings:
- antifibrinolytics (e.g. tranexamid acid)
- systemic hormone therapies
- levonorgestrel IUS (MIRENA®)
- transcervical endometrial resection/-ablation
- supracervical hysterectomy (LASH, abdominal)
- total hysterectomy

Hormonal therapies:
- progestagens (cyclic)
- progestagens (continuous)
- oral contraceptives cyclically or extended cycle (84/7 day-regimen) or continuous long-term application
- levonorgestrel IUS (MIRENA®)

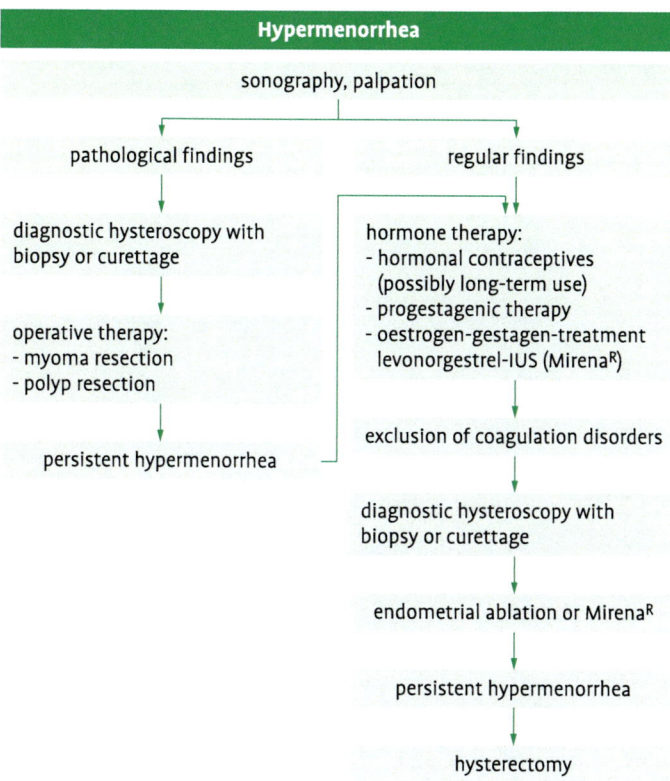

Fig. 7.35: Hypermenorrhea – diagnostic and therapeutic steps.

Table 7.15: Success rate of different treatments of hypermenorrhea.

Therapy	Reduction in bleeding intensity in %
Tranexamid acid (Cyklokapron®)	45
Long-term application of oral contraceptives	50
Progestagens (continuous)	87
MIRENA®	90
Endometrial ablation	80–90
LASH	95
Total hysterectomy	100

Note: A complete amenorrhea can only be achieved by a **total** hysterectomy (information of the patient!).

Aim of the endometrial ablation

Reduction in bleeding intensity with recurrent therapy-resistant recurrent hypermenorrheas.

Possibilities of endometrial ablation/-resection:

- 1. generation
  coagulation with the roller-ball-electrode
  - resection with the cutting loop
  - ND: YAG-laser
- 2. generation
  - hydrothermal ablation
  - bipolar electrode (NovaSure®)
  - microwave
  - uterine balloon techniques for the thermal coagulation of the endometrium (e.g. Thermachoice®)

Inclusion criteria for endometrial ablation:

- recurrent hypermenorrhea resistant to therapy (persistent for more than 1 year, and hormonal treatment without success)
- finished family planning!
- exclusion of complex and atypical endometrial hyperplasias and uterine cancer

- regular genital findings or small, solitary submucous myomas (diameter <3 cm) (sonography, hysteroscopy, histology)
- informed consent of the patient after extensive information about risks and benefits of the therapy
- uterine probe length <10 cm

Indications for endometrial ablation

- recurrent hypermenorrhea resistant to therapy
- perimenopausal bleeding disorders resistant to therapy
- bleeding disorders with coagulopathies and in patients undergoing long-term anticoagulant therapy
- anesthesiological risk group with contraindications for a hysterectomy
- therapy-resistant bleeding disorders during a postmenopausal hormone therapy
- bleeding disorders and endometrium hyperplasia during a tamoxifen treatment
- menstrual hygiene for patients seriously in need of nursing care

Note: An exact indication for the endometrial ablation is decisive for the prognosis.

Note: For patients with multiple myomas an endometrial ablation has only cosmetic effects and is in most of the cases not very efficient. In these cases the hysterectomy (if necessary, supracervical) remains the method of choice.

Information of the patient before endometrial ablation

- alternative to hormonal therapies (MIRENA®)
- alternative to hysterectomy (vaginal, LASH, LAVH, TLH)
- postoperative rate of amenorrheas approx. 35 %

- success rate (reduction of pathological bleedings): 80–90 % (depending on method and findings)
- failure rate: 10–20 %
- possible intraoperative complications (perforation, TUR-syndrome, secondary bleeding, infection)
- possible postoperative complications (haematometra, post-ablation-syndrome, pregnancies, recurrence, infections)
- necessity of additional contraception (if necessary, simultaneous laparoscopic tubal sterilisation or postoperative insertion of MIRENA®)

Note: The endometrial ablation is **no method of contraception.**

Endometrial ablation with pretreatment – diagnostic and therapeutic procedure

1. indication
2. vaginal sonography
3. outpatient hysteroscopy with biopsy or hysteroscopy with curettage
4. pretreatment for 4 to 8 weeks
5. alternatively: surgery in the early proliferative phase of the menstrual cycle (in most of the cases resection is necessary)
6. endometrial ablation or –resection
7. follow-up sonography and examination of the bleeding patterns after 3, 6 and 12 months and further annual follow-up

Note: A diagnostic hysteroscopy and biopsy are no longer necessary if the histological findings are regular after 6 months.

Endometrial ablation without pretreatment

With regular sonographic findings the endometrial ablation can be performed post menstruationem provided a resection with biopsy and adequate intraoperative histology are carried out, too.

Possibilities of pretreatment for endometrial ablation with the roller-ball-technique or the Nd-YAG-laser

- GnRH-analogues, 1 to 2 injections at intervals of 4 weeks (e.g. Enantone Gyn®, Zoladex®)
- progestagens (e.g. dienogest 4 mg/d), 4 to 6 weeks

In a prospective randomized comparative study a pretreatment with GnRH-analogues – one injection of the 4-weeks-effective GnRH-analogue Triptorelinacetate (Decapeptyl-Depot®) and a pretreatment with danazol (Winobanin® 600 mg/d for 4 weeks) – proved to be of advantage over a pretreatment with progestagens and a control group without pretreatment. This concerns the subjective assessment of the surgeon, the histology of the preoperative endometrium biopsy and the postoperative bleeding patterns.

Reference:

Römer, Th et al.: Hormonal premedication in endometrium ablation – results of a prospective comparative study. Zentralbl Gynakol 1996; 118: 291–4

Pretreatment for endometrial ablation

Note: Because of the short time of application side effects of the pretreatment play only a minor role.

The vaginal-sonographic measurement of the endometrium thickness is an indicator for the achieved suppression of the endometrium.

Vaginal sonography:

- optimal suppression of the endometrium thickness: thin
- sufficient suppression: double endometrium thickness <4 mm

Table 7.16: Pretreatment for endometrial ablation.

Advantages	Disadvantages
• better conditions (shorter duration of surgery) • easier scheduling of surgery • slightly increased rate of amenorrheas to be expected • use of coagulation techniques (e.g. roller ball) possible when histological findings are available	• increase in costs • possible side effects of hormone therapy • in most of the cases two surgeries necessary (2nd anaesthesia!): diagnostic hysteroscopy, then operative hysteroscopy

Note: The effect of the pretreatment on the rate of amenorrhea and on the necessity of secondary surgical interventions declines continuously after surgery.

Reference:

Sowter MC, Lethaby A, Singla A: Preoperative endometrial thinning agents before endometrial destruction for heavy menstrual bleeding. Cochrane Database Syst Rev 2000 (2) CD 001 124

Factors contributing to the success of the endometrial ablation

Better prognosis:
- age above 40
- pretreatment with GnRH-analogues and Danazol
- no dysmenorrhea ($\rightarrow$ adenomyosis score page 88)
- length of uterus <10 cm
- experienced surgeon

No influence on prognosis:
- additional simultaneous myoma resection (solitary submucous myomas <3 cm)
- technique (roller-ball-technique = resection technique = laser coagulation)

Note: The combination of the resection by cutting loop (anterior, posterior and lateral walls) and the roller-ball-coagulation (fundus, tubal corners) constitutes the gold standard of endometrial ablation because it unites the advantages of both methods.

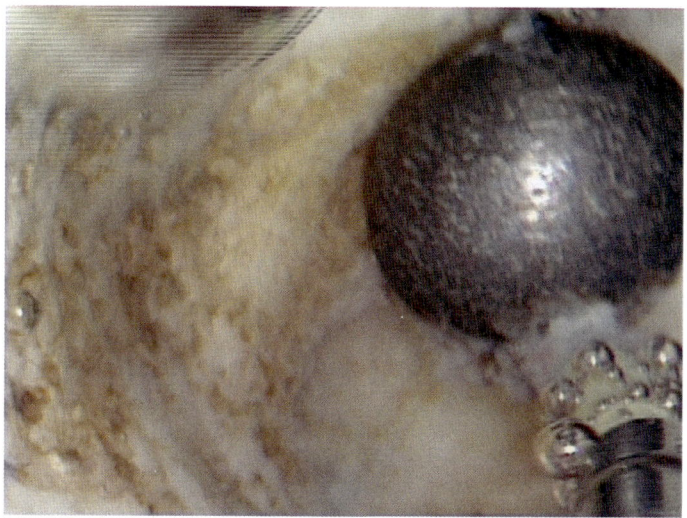

Fig. 7.36: Roller-ball-ablation (monopolar technique).

Table 7.17: Advantages and disadvantages of the endometrial ablation and -resection

	Endometrial ablation (roller-ball)	Endometrial resection (cutting loop)
intraoperative histology	none	yes
risk of perforation	lower	higher
intraoperative bleedings	minimal	considerably more
intraoperative view	good	made difficult by floating resectates
pretreatment	necessary	recommended

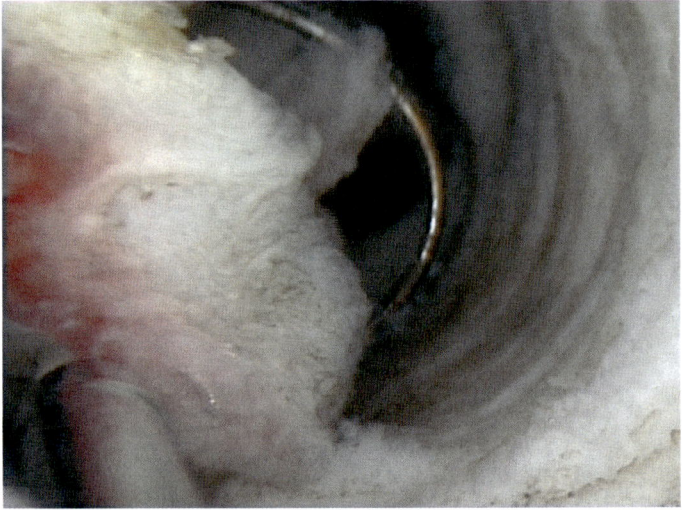

Fig. 7.37: Endometrial resection (monopolar technique).

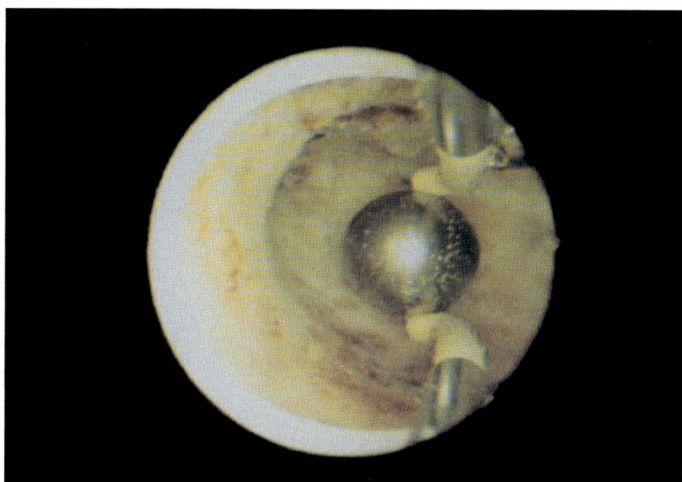

Fig. 7.38: Roller-ball-coagulation on the right lateral wall – endometrium sufficiently coagulated.

Note: The roller-ball-coagulation is most difficult on the anterior wall of the cavity because the intraoperative view is made difficult by build-up of air bubbles.

Practical advice: More frequent suction of the air bubbles and commencement of coagulation on the anterior wall!

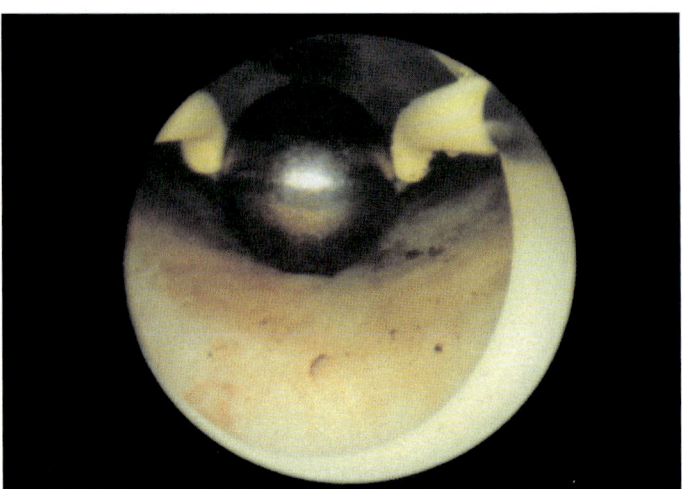

Fig. 7.39: Roller-ball-coagulation on the posterior wall of the cavity:
- posterior wall is completely coagulated, noticeable by the colour of the coagulated endometrium
- the ball rolls easily over the coagulated area without sinking into the endometrium

Note: A smooth rolling/movement of the electrode is a clear sign of a sufficient coagulation (2–3 mm into the myometrium)!

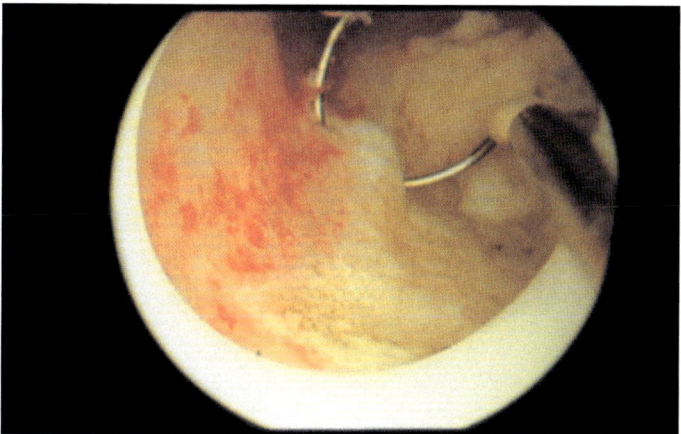

Fig. 7.40: Endometrial resection with the cutting loop:
- *on the left*: already resected endometrium (yellow – white)
- *on the right*: endometrium still to be removed (reddish)

Note: A complete resection of the endometrium and of parts of the myometrium (up to 2–4 mm) is necessary.

Cave: With resection in the tubal corners and in the fundal area there is a high risk of perforation!

Practical advice: In the tubal corners and in the fundal area a roller-ball-coagulation should be performed if possible.

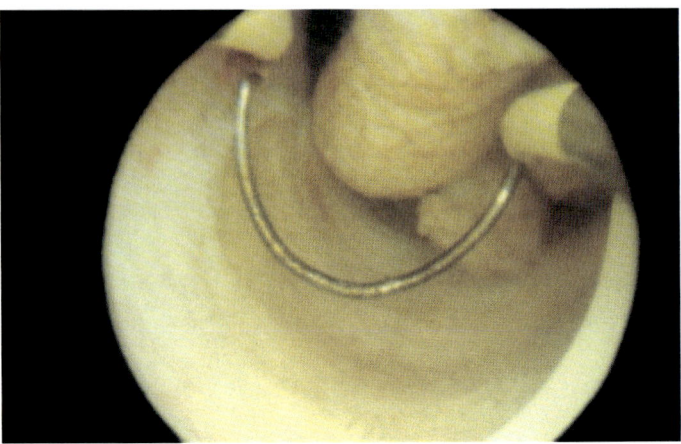

Fig. 7.41: Endometrial resection with the cutting loop – floating resectates obstruct the intraoperative view and have to be removed from time to time.

Note: The resectates should be removed by a blunt curette to avoid another damage of the coagulated areas.

Results and assessment of endometrial ablation

Table 7.18: Current data on long-term results of the endometrial ablation.

Author (year)	Follow-up	Patients	Rate of hysterectomy (%)	Success rate (%)
Boe-Engelsen (2006), Norway	4 –10 years	386	16.6	83.4
Fürst (2007), Denmark	10 years	120	22	78
Cooper (2001), Scotland	5 years	93	19	81
Litta (2006), Italy	6 –12 years	106	11.3	89.7
Own results	6 years	368	11.4	89.6

ACOG Practice Bulletin May 2007

LEVEL A: High rate of patient satisfaction after endometrial ablation – but it is still lower than after hysterectomy.

LEVEL B: Rate of hysterectomies after endometrial resection and alternative methods is 24% (follow- up 4 years)

Table 7.19: Comparison of the results of MIRENA and endometrial ablation (methods of the 1st generation).

Author	Year	Method of comparison	Patients [n/n]	Success rate (MIRENA®) (%)	Success rate (method of comparison) (%)
Crosignani	1997	endometrial resection	35/35	85	94
Römer	2000	endometrial ablation	15/15	73	93
Istre	2001	endometrial resection	30/29	67	90
Pellicano	2002	endometrial resection	41/41	70	85
Rauramo	2004	endometrial resection	30/29	63	76
Gupta	2006	endometrial resection	25/25	97	94

Table 7.20: Comparison MIRENA and endometrial ablation: Advantages and disadvantages.

	MIRENA®	Endometrial ablation
Initial bleeding disorder	yes (3–6 months)	no
Duration of therapy	5 years	possibly lifelong
Surgery with anaesthesia	no (only insertion)	yes
Success rate	70%	80%
Rate of amenorrhea	25%	35%
Reversible	yes	no
Finished family planning necessary	no	yes
Additional contraception necessary	no	yes (risk of 0.7%)
Alternative	endometrial ablation	hysterectomy

Note: When the family planning is not yet surely finished, the insertion of MIRENA should be given preference over the endometrial ablation. (information is compulsory!)

Table 7.21: Comparison of endometrial ablation/-resection and hysterectomy.

Endometrial ablation	Hysterectomy (TLH, LASH, vaginal)
organ-saving	organ loss
30% rate of amenorrhea	100% rate of amenorrhea
80–90% success rate	100% success rate
shorter time of surgery and anaesthesia	longer time of surgery and anaesthesia
shorter stay in hospital	longer stay in hospital
shorter return-to-work time	longer return-to-work time
no blood transfusions (0%)	blood transfusions may be necessary (1–3%)
less antibiotics (5%)	more antibiotics (60%)
less analgetics (50%)	more analgetics (100%)

Specific complications of the endometrial ablation

- haematometra
- endometritis (▶ page 113)
- post-ablation syndrome
- first symptoms of an endometrial cancer may be obscured
- pregnancies
- recurrences

Haematometra

The risk of a haematometra is very low (<1%). It can also occur after the use of a method of the 2nd generation (after Thermachoice®: risk of 0.6–3%).

The haematometra can be treated conservatively (cervical dilatation and, if necessary, re-ablation), but because of the risk of recurrence in most of the cases a hysterectomy is preferred.

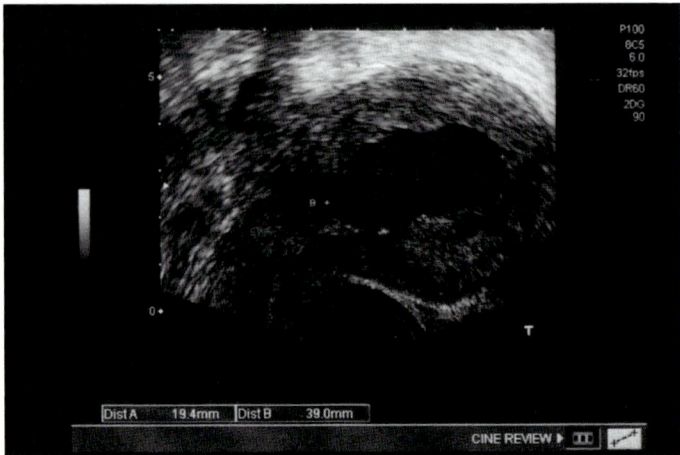

Fig. 7.42: Sonographic findings of a haematometra – 12 months after endometrial ablation.
Causes of the haematometra:
- coagulation – too deep into the cervical area
- secondary cervical infection with cervical occlusion

Note: During the endometrial ablation the cervix has to be spared from coagulation or resection because of the risk of a later haematometra.

Literature also reports of a secondary manifestation of a haematometra after the beginning of a cyclic postmenopausal HT. With lower abdominal pain during postmenopausal HT after endometrial ablation this should be considered in differential diagnostics.

Reference:

Dwyer N, Fox R, Mills M: Haematometra caused by hormone replacement therapy after endometrial resection. Lancet 1991; 338: 1205

Note: When a haematometra occurs after endometrial ablation an ectopic pregnancy should also be excluded.

Post-ablation syndrome

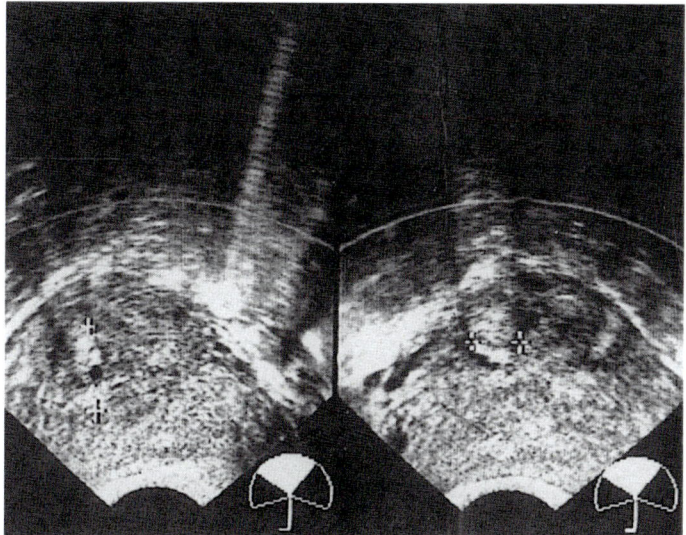

Fig. 7.43: Sonographic findings of a cavity filled with liquid in the right tubal corner – 18 months after endometrial ablation.

Note: The post-ablation syndrome is a long-term complication of the endometrial ablation.

Symptoms
Increasing pelvic pain (unilateral or bilateral tension pain), usually 12–36 months after endometrial ablation, sometimes also manifestation as a haematosalpinx.

Diagnostics
- symptoms
- target sonography of the tubal corners

Note: A post-ablation syndrome has only little clinical relevance (<1%). Some publications mention an incidence of up to 10% with specific diagnostics.

Reference:

McClausland AM, McClausland VM: Frequency of symptomatic cornual hematometra and postablation tubal sterilization syndrome after total rollerball endometrial ablation: a 10-year follow-up. Am J Obstet Gynecol 2002; 186: 1274–80

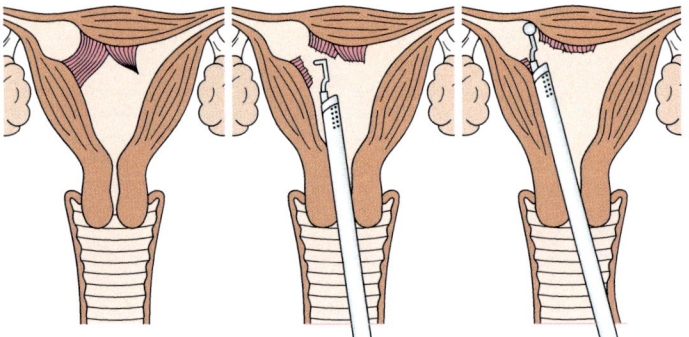

Fig. 7.44: Organ-retaining management of a post-ablation syndrome.
1. sonographic diagnostics
2. intrauterine adhesiolysis with resection needle with simultaneous abdominal sonography to open the cavity
3. second coagulation in this area with the little roller-ball

Note: The conservative therapy of the post-ablation syndrome is possible. However, it should be performed by a surgeon experienced in hysteroscopy and always with simultaneous sonographic control.

Practical advice: In this case, however, a hysterectomy should be preferred to organ-retaining therapy because of the recurrence risk.

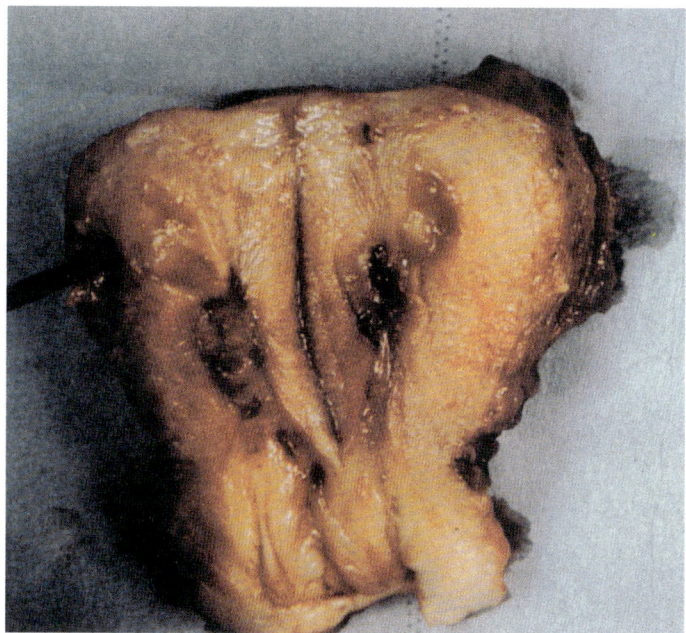

Fig. 7.45: Hysterectomy specimen of a patient with post-ablation syndrome; 12 months after endometrial ablation (picture: R. Campo, Leuven/Belgium).

Note: A hysterectomy is especially indicated for bilateral post-ablation syndromes. Before surgery the patients should be informed about this potential long-term complication.

Endometrial carcinoma after endometrial ablation

Problem:
possible delay of the diagnostics of endometrial carcinomas by missing first symptom: bleeding caused by intrauterine adhesions after endometrial ablation.

However,

- largest part of the endometrium is coagulated or resected (hypothetical risk reduction!)
- the endometrial resection covers early carcinomas which have not been removed by repeated abrasions. Literature refers to case studies regarding an early diagnostics of endometrial carcinomas or stromal sarcomas by endometrial resection.

Note: Essential for the exclusion of a complex or atypical hyperplasia and of carcinomas is a thorough pre-diagnostics. For patients with risk factors for an endometrial carcinoma the endometrium biopsy is not sufficient for pre-diagnostics.

Advantage of endometrial resection:
An exact intraoperative histology can be obtained. For that reason with all unclear endometrial findings this method is to be preferred to roller-ball endometrial ablation and other coagulation methods.

Postmenopausal hormonal therapy after transcervical endometrial ablation

- In 70% of the patients histological residual endometrium is found (also in cases of a postoperative amenorrhea).

  Note: After an endometrial ablation patients are to be treated for postmenopausal hormonal therapy the same way as patients with a uterus.

- The administration of progestagen to protect the endometrium is compulsory (continuous or cyclic)! Recommended is continuous HT or the administration of tibolone (Liviella®).
- In patients with therapy-resistant bleeding disorders during a cyclic hormone therapy a continuous HT after endometrial ablation can result in an almost 100% rate of amenorrhea.

Table 7.22: HT after endometrial ablation.

	ET (2 mg oestradiol)	HT (2 mg oestradiol + 1 mg NETA)
Patients	31	31
Endometrial hyperplasia without atypias	6	0
Proliferative endometrium	8	0
Bleeding rate and endometrium thickness	higher	–

Reference:

Istre O, Holm-Nielsen P, Bourne T et al.: Hormone replacement therapy after transcervical resection of the endometrium. Obstet Gynecol 1996; 88: 767–70

Note: A monotherapy with oestrogen after endometrial ablation results in endometrial hyperplasia and thus in increased bleeding rates.

Postoperative pregnancies after transcervical endometrial ablation

- risk by residual endometrium; implantation possible
- recommendation: simultaneous laparoscopic tubal sterilization in premenopausal patients with consideration of benefit and risk
- risk of postoperative pregnancy 0,24–0,7 %

One case study even reports of a pregnancy rate of 5.2 % (3/58) after the balloon-method.

Reference:

Gervaise A, de Tayrac R, Fernandez H: Contraceptive information after endometrial ablation. Fertil Steril 2005; 84: 1746–7

Note: Even after the use of a method of the second generation contraception is necessary.

The English-speaking literature reports of more than 74 pregnancies after endometrial ablation until 2006.

Reference:

Lo JS, Dickersgill A: Pregnancy after endometrial ablation: English literature review and case report. J Minim Invasive Gynecol 2006; 13: 88–91

Problems:
- pregnancy often diagnosed very late because patient suffers from hypo- or amenorrhea
- complications during pregnancy and delivery (placenta accreta or increta, intrauterine retardation)

Case studies also report of tubal pregnancies or cervical pregnancies after endometrial ablation.

Additionally, 2 cases of maternal death after endometrial ablation were reported.

The review of 70 pregnancies after endometrial ablation shows the high rate of complications.

Table 7.23: Outcome of 70 pregnancies after endometrial ablation.

31 pregnancies with high risk of complications	
Rate of premature deliveries	42%
Placenta adherens	26%
Small for gestation	39%
Caesarean sections	71%

Reference:

Hare AA, Olah KS: Pregnancy following endometrial ablation: a review article. J Obstet Gynecol 2005; 25: 108–14

Note: The endometrial ablation is no method of contraception. Premenopausal patients must be informed about that. Instead, the simultaneous tubal sterilization should be recommended.

Note: The insertion of a levonorgestrel IUS (MIRENA®) immediately after surgery is an alternative option of contraception after endometrial ablation. Moreover, it offers further advantages to the patient.

MIRENA® after endometrial ablation

Advantages:
- secure contraception (no additional contraception necessary)
- higher rate of amenorrhea (almost 100 %)
- co-treatment of dysmenorrhea (with adenomyosis and endometriosis)

Disadvantages:
- higher costs (in most of the cases no coverage of the costs by the health insurance providers)
- change of MIRENA® necessary after 5 years (?)

Table 7.24: Comparative studies of endometrial ablation (EA) with and without postoperative insertion of MIRENA®.

Author	Year	Patients n/n	Rate of amenorrhea	
			EA with MIRENA®	EA without MIRENA®
Römer	1997	13/13	92 %	54 %
Kreuz/Römer	2005	66/102	79 %	36 %
Maia	2003	53/42*	100 %	9 %

*) patients with adenomyosis

References:

Römer T: A prospective study for a combined hysteroscopic-local hormonal therapy of recurrent refractory hypermenorrheas. Geburtsh Frauenheilk 1997; 57: 614–6

Kreuz S: Bleeding patterns after endometrium ablation with and without progestagen-IUS. Inaugural-Dissertation, Medizinische Fakultät der Universität zu Köln, 2005

Maia H, Haltez A, Coelho G et al.: Insertion of MIRENA after endometrial resection in patients with adenomyosis. J Am Assoc Gyneco
Laparosc 2003; 10: 512–6

Recurrences of the endometrial ablation (adenomyosis)

Almost all recurrences are caused by an adenomyosis uteri, which
therapeutically may only be temporarily influenced by the endometrial ablation.

Own results:
- 42 hysterectomies after 368 endometrial ablations (11.4%)

Histological results of the hysterectomy specimen:
- 40 adenomyosis
- 2 leiomyomas

Note: The leading clinical symptom of the adenomyosis is **dysmenorrhea.**

Note: The indication for a repeated endometrial ablation should
be very carefully set because most of the recurrences are caused
by an adenomyosis. Therefore second surgical interventions do
not promise any long-term success of therapy.

Most frequent reason for treatment failure
of the endometrial ablation: adenomyosis

So far adenomyosis has been mostly diagnosed on the hysterectomy specimen. The preoperative diagnostics of an adenomyosis is
difficult. In these cases an adenomyosis-score including anamnestic, clinical and sonographic data can be helpful.

Table 7.25: Adenomyosis-score according to Römer.

Feature	0 points	1 point	2 points
Meno- or metrorrhagia	none	slight: Hb $\geq$7.4 mmol/l; only hypermenorrhea (coagula in menstrual blood, >4–5 sanitary pads/d) or only permanent bleeding (>7/d)	severe: Hb <7.4 mmol/l; hypermenorrhea + permanent bleeding
Dysmenorrhea	none	slight: no analgetic medication	severe: analgesics, limited quality of life
Uterus probe length	very small or very big uterine cavity: <5.5 cm; >9 cm	moderately diminished or enlarged uterine cavity: 5.5–6 cm; 8–9 cm	uterine cavity of normal size: 6–7.5 cm
Thickened myometrium (shown by sonography)	none	asymmetrical hyperplasia	symmetrical hyperplasia
Areas in the myometrium that do not reflecting echo (sonography)	none	heterogeneous region in the myometrium with areas not reflecting echo	several heterogeneous regions in the myometrium with areas not reflecting echo
Pregnancies	none	1	$\geq$2
Curettages	none	1	$\geq$2

Table 7.26: Adenomyosis-score and clinical consequences.

Score	Adenomyosis probability	Recommendation
<6	7%	well suited for endometrial ablation
6–10	44%	endometrial ablation possible
>10	100%	MIRENA® or hysterectomy

Note: With a score of more than 10 the endometrial ablation cannot be recommended.

Note: MRI-diagnostics of adenomyosis is possible. However, it is a very cost-intensive examination.

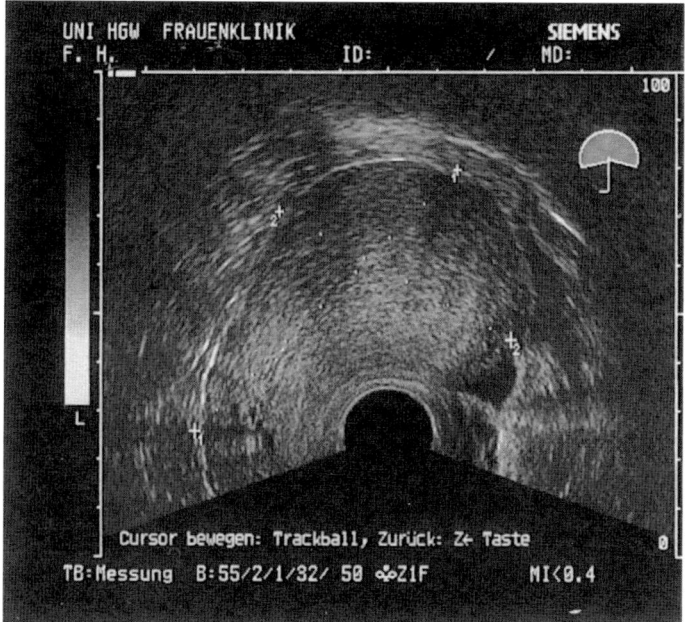

Fig. 7.46: Preoperative sonographic findings in a patient with the question: endometrial ablation because of recurrent hyper- and dysmenorrhea.

Suspicion: adenomyosis

Decision: vaginal hysterectomy

Histology: confirmation of the diagnosis adenomyosis

Sonographic evidence:
1. thickening of the myometrium (growth of the uterus)
2. irregular echo-free structures in the myometrium

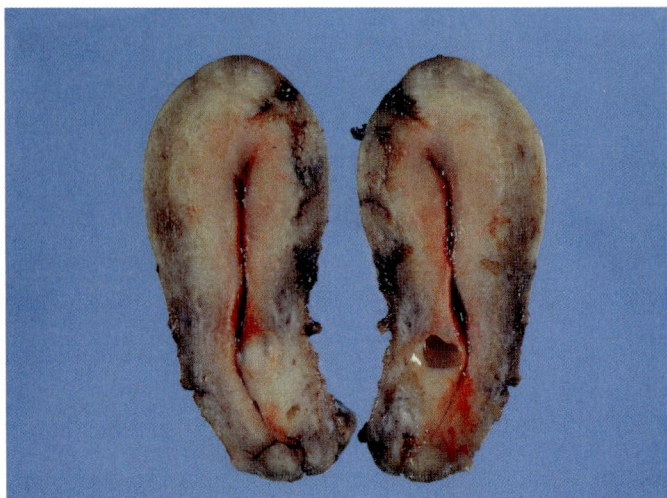

Fig. 7.47: Hysterectomy specimen 9 months after endometrial ablation with persistent hyper- and dysmenorrhea (histology: adenomyosis).

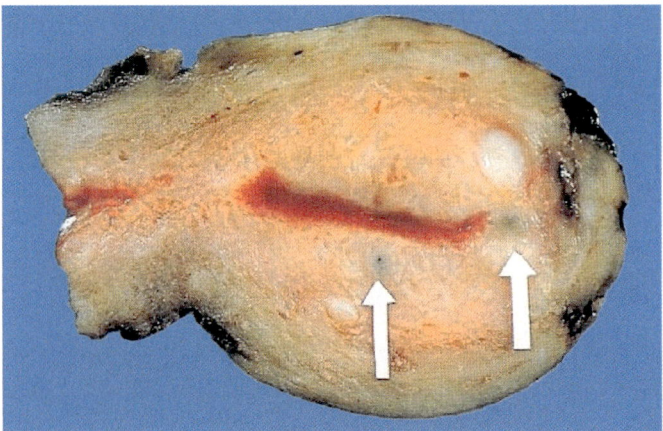

Fig. 7.48: Hysterectomy specimen with adenomyosis.

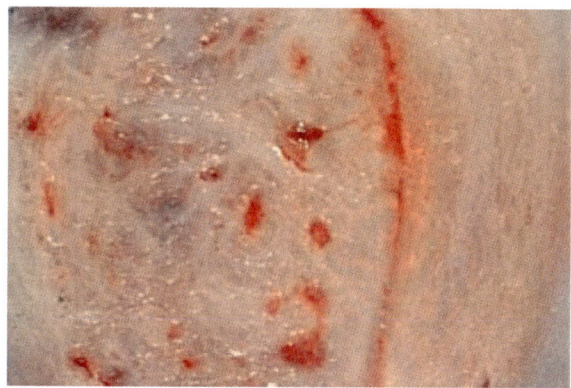

Fig. 7.49: Section preparation of adenomyosis.

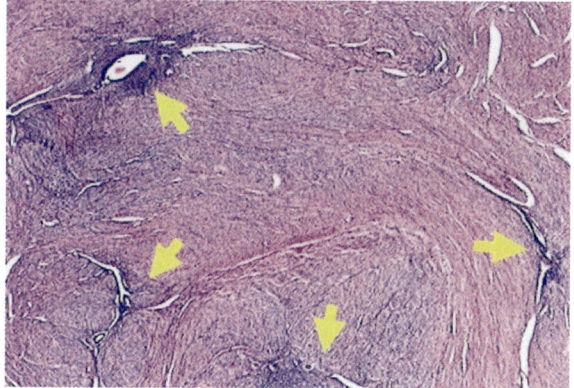

Fig. 7.50: Histological findings of an adenomyosis uteri.
Histological characteristics:
- endometrial glands
- cytogenic stroma
- reactive myometrial hyperplasia

I thank Assistant Professor Dr. Mellin of the Institute of Pathology Cologne-Lindenthal for the kind permission to use the histological pictures.

7.6 Alternative techniques of endometrial ablation

In Germany only two methods of the Second-Generation-Methods have established themselves in the medium term:
1. Uterine balloon therapy system (Thermachoice®)
2. Bipolar coagulation with NovaSure® ("gold-plated mesh")

Note: The Second-Generation-Methods are coagulation methods. For that reason preoperative **histological** diagnostics of bleeding disorders is necessary (similar to the procedure before a roller-ball-ablation).

Uterine balloon therapy system (Thermachoice®)

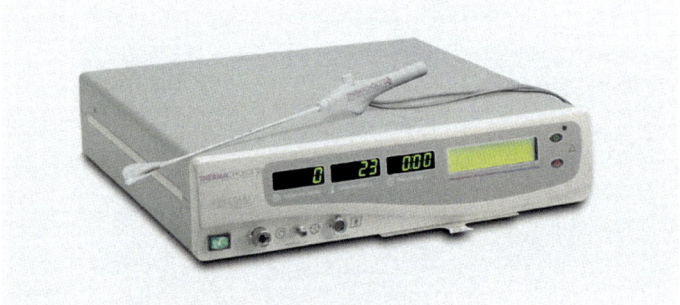

Fig. 7.51: Thermachoice®-catheter with generator.

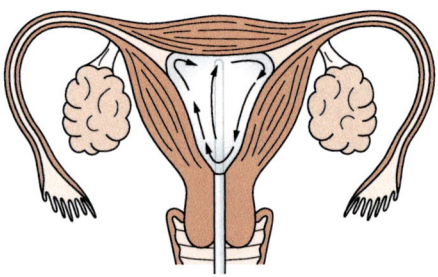

Fig. 7.52: Thermachoice®-catheter in the cavum uteri.

Fig. 7.51 is published with the kind permission of Ethicon ltd, Norderstedt.

Procedure of the uterine balloon therapy system (Thermachoice®)

- insertion of a thin disposable catheter 4.5 mm outer diameter) into the cavum uteri
- expansion of the balloon with fluid (5–15 ml, max 30 ml)
- activation of the heating element up to an initial pressure of 160–180 mmHg (do not exceed a pressure of 200 mmHg!)
- duration of treatment – 8 min: fluid in the balloon is heated and circulates
- at the end of the treatment: remove fluid from the balloon and remove catheter

Table 7.27: Comparative studies balloon therapy system versus endometrial ablation/-resection and long-term results.

Methods (author)	Follow-up	Patients	Success rate
Balloon therapy system Roller-ball (Meyer et al. 1998)	12 months	239	80.2% 84.3%
Balloon therapy system Roller-ball (van Zon-Rabelink et al. 2004)	24 months	137	80.0% 75.0%
Balloon therapy system Endometrial resection (Gervaise et al. 1999)	12 months	147	83.0% 76.0%
Balloon therapy system (Ahonkallio et al. 2008) Long-term study	6 years	190	76.0% (16 hysterectomy)

Comparison of the uterine balloon therapy system (Thermachoice®) and the electrosurgical endometrial ablation

Advantages:
- can be performed with local anesthesia (also in patients suffering from cervical stenosis)
- well-suited for risk patients

Disadvantages:
- rate of amenorrhea slightly lower than after endometrial ablation or with NovaSure®
- not applicable with additional bleeding disorders (myomas, polyps) or with uterus malformations
- contra-indicated after Caesarean section or myoma enucleation
- more frequent postoperative side-effects 91.8%: cramps, lower abdominal pain and 23.9%: nausea and emesia)
- in most of the cases no coverage by the statutory health insurers

Note: Even if there is only a slight uterus malformation, there is an increased risk of a post-ablation syndrome caused by insufficient coagulation of the tubal corners.

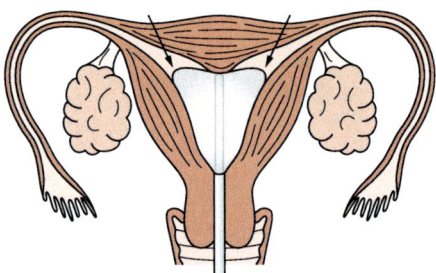

Fig. 7.53: Risk of the development of a post-ablation syndrome when using the balloon therapy system with a uterus arcuatus.

NovaSure® endometrial ablation

Compared with endometrial ablation, the NovaSure® method has the advantage of a higher rate of amenorrhea and a significantly shorter duration of surgery.

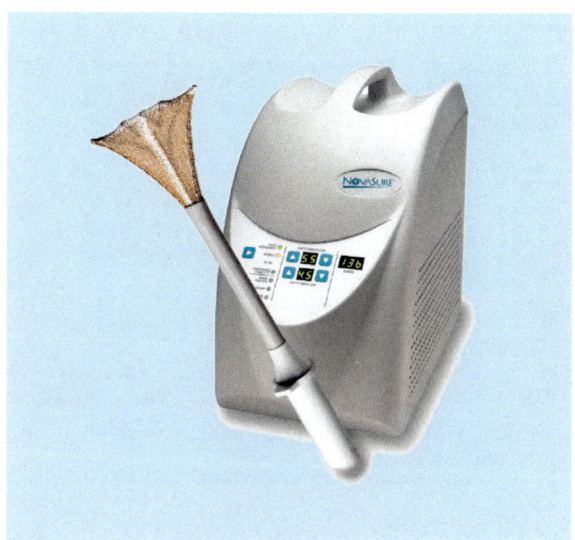

Fig. 7.54: NovaSure®-applicator

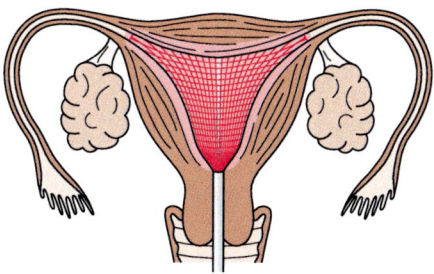

Fig. 7.55: NovaSure®-mesh in the cavum uteri

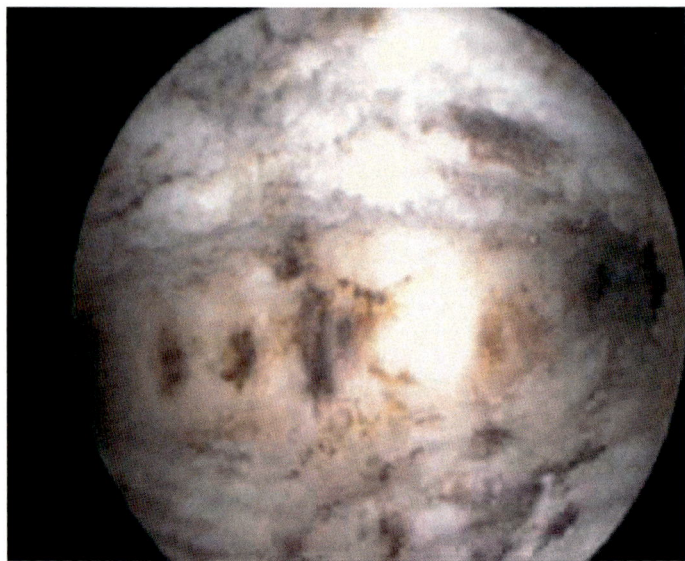

Fig. 7.56: Final findings with coagulation of the cavum uteri after application of NovaSure®.

Figures 7.54 and 7.56 are published with kind permission of Hologic Germany Ltd, Frankfurt/Main.

Table 7.28: Comparison of the results of NovaSure® and electrosurgical endometrial ablation after 24 months (randomized prospective study).

	NovaSure	Endometrial ablation
Patients (n)	147	102
Age (years)	39.8	41.0
Bleeding pattern after 24 months		
Amenorrhea	53.7%	32.4%
Spottings	36.7%	11.8%
Hypomenorrhea	4.0%	40.2%
Eumenorrhea	4.0%	4.9%
Hypermenorrhea	1.3%	2.0%
Hysterectomy	0	8.8%

Reference:

Römer T, Socko P, Kreuz G: High frequency ablation versus transcervical endometrial resection-prospective comparison study of treatment of recurrent hypermenorrhea. Frauenarzt 2010; 51: 942–948

Table 7.29: Advantages and disadvantages of the endometrial abla-tion/-resection compared with the NovaSure® method.

	Endometrial ablation/-resection (gold standard)	NovaSure®
Rate of amenorrhea (%)	30–35	55–75
Success rate (%)	80–85	95–98
Rate of hysterectomy (%)	10–20	0–5
Intraoperative histology	yes	no
Pretreatment	with surgery post menstruationem – not necessary	not necessary
Risk of perforation	low	almost completely excluded
Success dependent on menstrual cycle?	yes	no
Coverage of costs	yes	no general cost coverage of the material costs (statutory health insurers)
Risks of surgery	dependent on surgeon	independent of surgeon
Application with submucous myomas	possible (+ myoma resection)	not possible
Application with uterus malformations	possible	not possible

Table 7.30: Comparison Mirena® and endometrial ablation (method of the second generation).

Author	Year	Method of comparison	Patients n/n	Success rate (Mirena®) %	Success rate (method of comparison) %
Soysal	2002	Thermachoice	36/36	69	70
Henshaw	2002	Microwave	23/39	75	75
Barrington	2003	Thermachoice	23/21	90	90
Busfield	2006	Thermachoice	40/39	72	74
Tam	2006	Thermachoice	22/22	67	100
Shaw	2007	Thermachoice	33/33	79	87

Note: Before performing second-generation-methods the patient should be informed about an alternative therapy with Mirena®.

Significance of the second-generation-methods

When applying these methods the following potential pros and cons should be weighed up:
1. **Thermachoice**® – local anesthesia possible, with potential un-favourable postoperative results
2. **NovaSure**® – higher rate of amenorrhea and higher costs

The costs of both methods (net prices):
- Thermachoice®:   579 Euro per catheter
- NovaSure®:   750 Euro per applicator

should be weighed up with their advantages and disadvantages against the gold standard method.

Note: Insufficient experience of the surgeon should not be an indication for the application of a second-generation-method.

Table 7.31: Comparison of the techniques of the endometrial ablation (Cochrane-analysis).

	Second-generation-method	OR
Duration of surgery	shorter (15 min)	–
Local anesthesia	more frequent	8.3
Technical errors	more frequent	4.2
Complications	less frequent	TUR-syndrome 0.13 perforation of the uterus 0.21 injury of the cervix 0.12 haematometra 0.25
Side effects	more frequent (nausea, cramps of the uterus)	2.3

Reference:

Lethaby A, Hickey M, Garry R: Endometrial destruction techniques for heavy menstrual bleeding. Cochrane Database Syst Rev 2002 (2) CD001501

7.7 Special features of the bipolar surgical technique

With the development of the bipolar technique the scope of the operative hysteroscopy expands and the procedure gets even safer.

The decisive advantage of the bipolar hysteroscopy is that it can be performed without an electrolyte-free solution (Sorbitol-Mannitol-solution). Instead, Ringer's or saline solution can be used.

This results in lower costs of the distending medium.

Note: For risk situations (e.g. myomas of grade 2/ESGE) the bipolar hysteroscopy is the current method of choice because of a reduced rate of complications.

Bipolar techniques in the intrauterine surgery

Note: Bipolar techniques gain increasingly in importance in the operative hysteroscopy.

Bipolar techniques in hysteroscopy can contribute to solving some problems of intrauterine surgery and to increasing the safety of the patient.

Preferred indications for the bipolar surgical technique:
- myomas grade 2/ESGE
- large myomas (>4cm)

Main advantages of the bipolar myoma resection:
- avoidance of the TUR-syndrome, e.g. electrolyte shifts
- avoidance of second or third surgeries resulting thereof

Note: Even with the use of Ringer's solution an overload should be avoided. The fluid deficit should not exceed 3 l! Even higher caution is necessary with anaesthesiological risk groups.

Necessary technical requirements for the bipolar technique compared with monopolar resection:
- bipolar hysteroresectoscope (lenses can still be used) (▶ page 14)
- bipolar cable
- high frequency unit with bipolar programme (Autocon II 400) (▶ page 10)
- bipolar electrodes (reusable) (▶ page 15)
- Ringer's solution as distending medium (▶ page 17)

Note: When purchasing new equipment nowadays the bipolar technique should be preferred because it is going to completely replace the monopolar technique in the future.

Note: The bipolar hysteroscopic procedure is the same as the monopolar one.

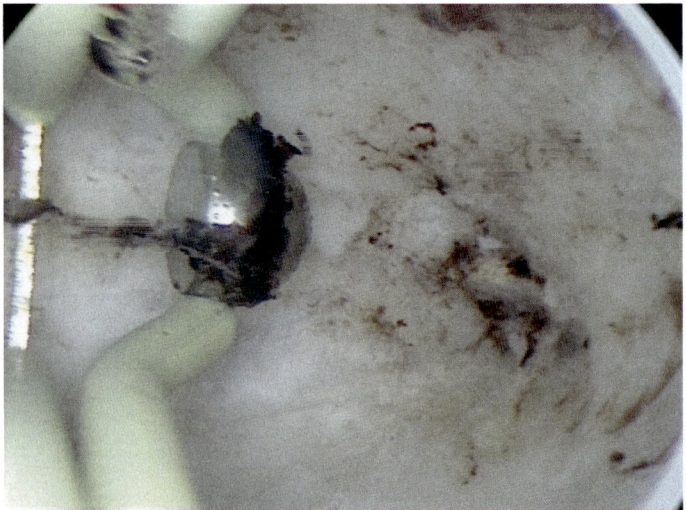

Fig. 7.57: Endometrial ablation with the bipolar coagulation electrode.

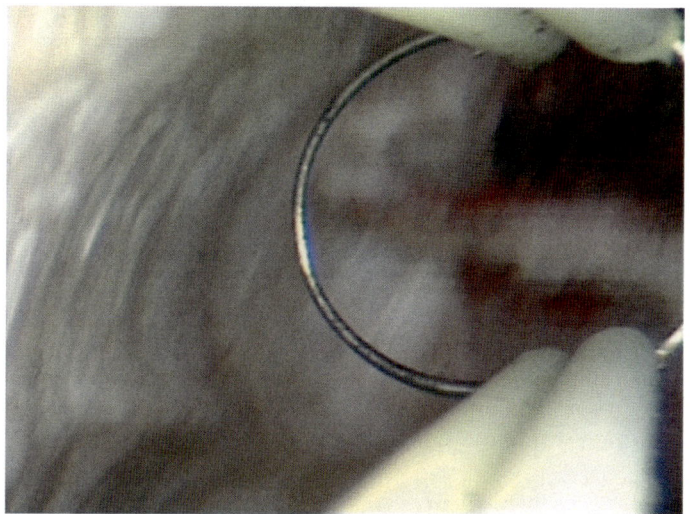

Fig. 7.58: Bipolar endometrial resection.

Bipolar myoma resection

52 myoma resections (2006–2008) Academic Hospital Cologne-Weyertal

20 myomas – grade 1

32 myomas – grade 2

- resection during first surgery possible in 50 of the 52 patients
- second resection only in 2 patients with myomas >8 cm because of lack of intraoperative view
- average weight of the myomas: 40 g (20–120g)

Note: With the bipolar technique second surgery can be almost completely avoided. Second surgery with very large submucous myomas is often only necessary with lack of intraoperative view because of increased bleedings.

Table 7.32: Comparison of mono- and bipolar surgical techniques exemplified by the resection of a myoma grade 2/ESGE.

	Monopolar resection	Bipolar resection
Equipment	standard	additional equipment
Distending medium	Sorbitol-Mannitol-solution	Ringer's solution
Danger of TUR-syndrome	high	no
Costs distending medium (e.g. consumption of 3 l)	4.83 Euro	4.75 Euro
Level of training of surgeon	no difference	no difference
Second surgery	frequent	rare
Results with large myoma grade 2	after first surgery: about 60 % success	after first surgery: about 95 % success

In infertile patients the application of the bipolar technique (e.g. with the septum dissection or the intrauterine adhesiolysis) may hypothetically lead to a slight thermal damage of the surrounding tissue (endometrium) (lack of data!).

Note: Also in problem situations with increased vascularisation of intracavitary findings or in the endometrium (e.g. residual placenta) the bipolar hysteroscopy is a safer method than the monopolar technique.

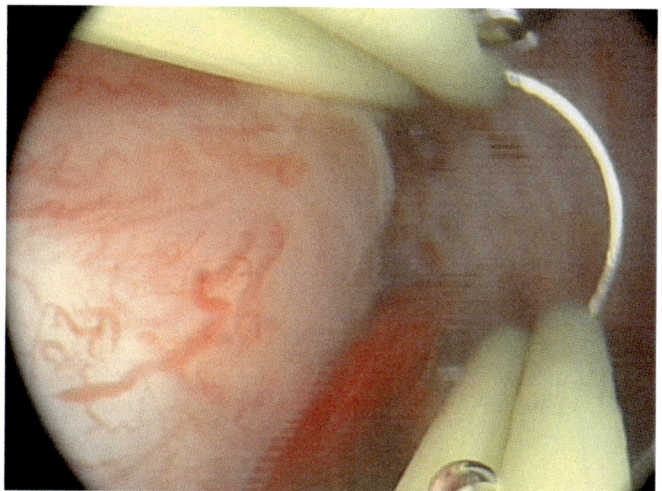

Fig. 7.59: Start of the bipolar myoma resection.

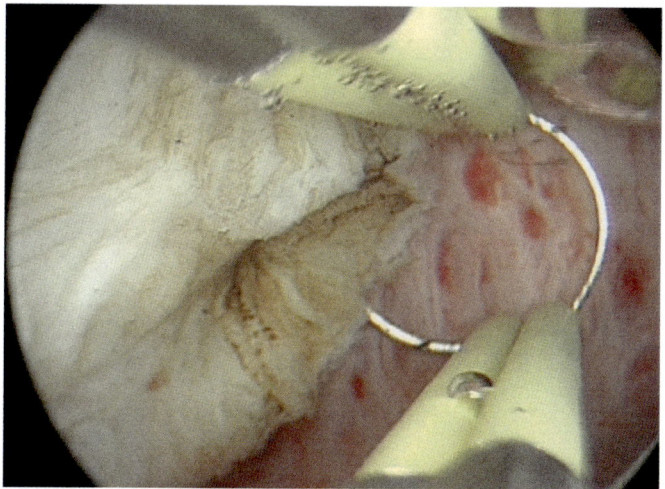

Fig. 7.60: Bipolar myoma resection.

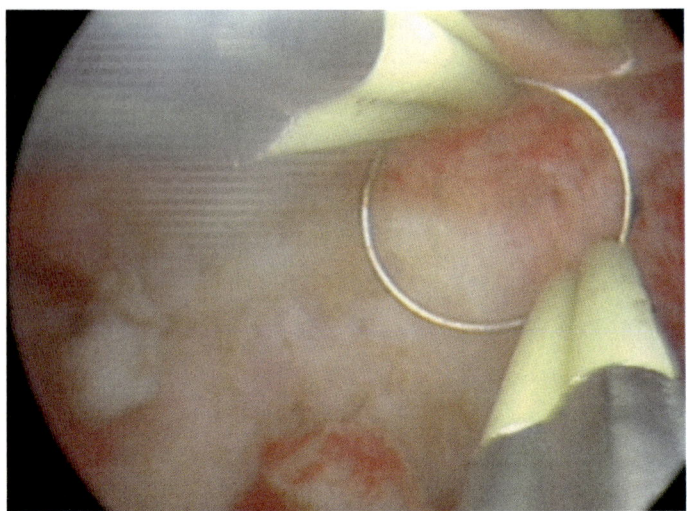

Fig. 7.61: Final findings after bipolar myoma resection.

Advantages of bipolar hysteroscopy:
- avoidance of TUR-syndrome by use of Ringer's solution
- longer time for surgery possible resulting in reduced need for second operations
- optimised, controlled power output for all tissue structures – resulting in
- surgery of infertile patients, treating the endometrium with care
- optimised power level leading to a resection with less bleedings – post-coagulation is only necessary in rare cases

8 General complications of operative hysteroscopy: management and prevention

Possible complications of the operative hysteroscopy:
- perforation with injury of other pelvic organs
- bleeding
- infection
- TUR-syndrome
- burns
- air embolism

8.1 Perforation

Note: The highest risk of perforation exists with electrosurgical interventions with the cutting loop and with intrauterine adhesiolyses.

Safety aspects

With the resection of myomas with an intramural part the sonographic distance between myoma and serosa should be at least 8 mm (▶ page 54).

Note: With a complete intramural myoma a simultaneous check by abdominal sonography is recommended.

Note: With intrauterine adhesiolyses of grades III and IV/ESGE a simultaneous sonography or laparoscopy should be performed if necessary.

Note: On least suspicion of perforation – immediate laparoscopy, because otherwise risk of electrosurgical lesion of neighbouring organs (especially the bowel). If a thermal lesion of neighbouring organs cannot be excluded for sure, a laparotomy is justified.

Note: With postoperative lower abdominal symptoms (even if after some time) undetected perforations of the uterus should always be considered by differential diagnostics.

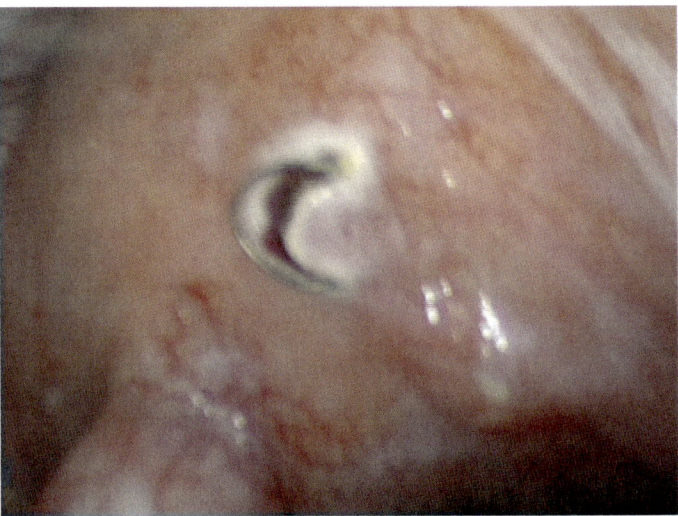

Fig. 8.1: Perforation with the cutting loop without lesion of the neighbouring organs.

Note: In most of the cases the laparoscopy is only useful in the diagnostics of a perforation, not for its prevention! For the prevention of a perforation the simultaneous abdominal sonography outperforms a laparoscopy.

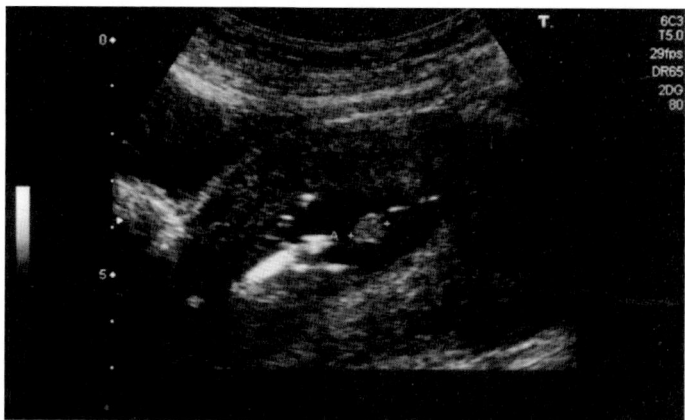

Fig. 8.2: Abdominal sonography with the resection of a submucous myoma.

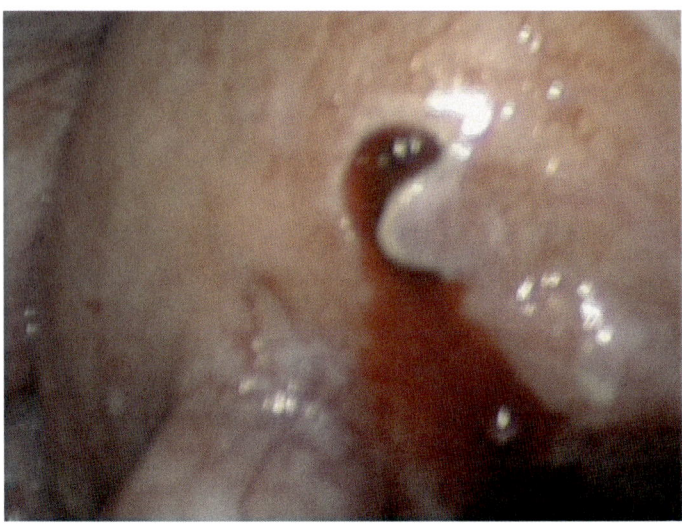

Fig. 8.3: Bleeding from the perforation wound requires stopping of haemorrhage by coagulation or suture.

Note: After a perforation the patient should always be administered antibiotics. Additionally, close and frequent clinical and laboratory postoperative monitoring is necessary.

8.2 Intra- and postoperative bleedings

● most frequent after myoma resections

Cave: **Do not** misinterpret outflowing distending medium diluted with blood as severe secondary bleeding.

Management of secondary bleeding:
● contraction agent i.v. (dosage ► page 53), if necessary, repeated injection
● intracavitary insertion of a Foley-catheter (blocking for 24 hours)

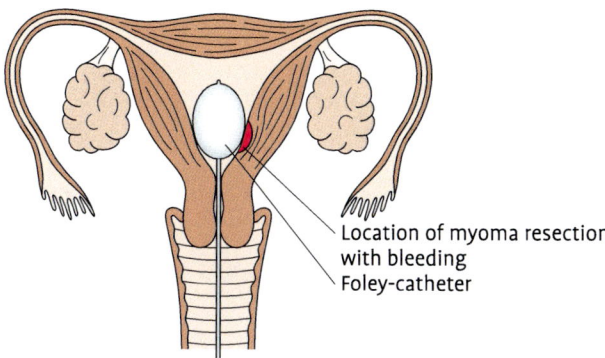

Location of myoma resection
with bleeding
Foley-catheter

Fig. 8.4: Insertion of a Foley-catheter for the treatment of severe bleedings after myoma resection.

Preventive measures:
- diligent coagulation of the visible bleeding focus at the end of surgery (especially in the area of the vascular supply of the myoma)

Note: At the end of surgery intrauterine bleeding foci only become visible after an intrauterine reduction of pressure. Then a targeted coagulation is possible, either by cutting loop or by switch to the roller-ball electrodes.

8.3 Infections

- theoretical risk of ascending infection
- with preoperative exclusion of colpitis, cervicitis and endometritis the risk is very low
- in risk patients (immunosuppressed patients, diabetic patients) an antibiotic prophylaxis is recommended.
- special cases of necrotizing endometritis, pyometra and tubo-ovarian abscesses are described in the literature. However, these may also occur after the second-generation-method of the endometrial ablation.

Preoperative diagnostics with clinical abnormalities:
- exclusion of colpitis (native preparation, microbiology)
- preoperative laboratory (leucocytes, CRP)
- palpation (exclusion of adnexitis)
- sonography (exclusion of tubo-ovarian abscesses or pyometra)

Note: The peripoperative antibiotic prophylaxis with the operative hysteroscopy is an individual decision. A compulsory antibiotic prophylaxis is not necessary! However, in risk patients, or longer intrauterine interventions or with complications an antibiotic prophylaxis is recommended.

8.4 TUR-syndrome (Transurethral resection syndrome)

Synonyms:
- fluid overload syndrome (FOS)
- overinfusion syndrome
- hysteroscopy syndrome
- transcervical resection syndrome (TCRS)
- absorption syndrome

Definition:
Increased intravascular absorption of an electrolyte-free hypotonic distending medium causing extra- and intracellular disorders in the electrolyte and water metabolism, which result in clinical symptoms

Causes:
- incision into a vessel (mainly with resection methods, especially with myoma resection)
- inflow of the medium into the circulation, caused by intrauterine pressure
- intracellular water shift

Safety aspects:
- pressure and flow control by a hysteromat during hysteroscopy
- permanent fluid balance
- with borderline cases (fluid deficit >700 ml) – intraoperative determination of electrolytes (sodium)
- with fluid deficit >1,000 ml: break surgery off or cut it short

Note: Bipolar hysteroscopies also require a fluid balance to avoid the isotonic overload of the patient. With a fluid deficit from >40 ml/kg body weight/h (within one hour in patients without cardiovascular problems) surgery should be cut short.

Clinical symptoms of the TUR-syndrome

In patients under anaesthesia the diagnosis is mainly based on **cardiopulmonary symptoms**:
- impaired gas exchange (i.e. decrease in oxygen saturation), pulmonary oedema
- increase in ventilation pressure, decrease in pulmonary compliance
- increase in central venous pressure
- circulatory dysregulation (hypertonia, later hypotonia)
- vena cava superior syndrome
- cardiac decompensation, arrhythmia,
- bradycardia
- polyuria

In the awake patient **central venous symptoms** are of more importance:
- restlessness
- frequent yawning (often a first sign)
- confusion, disorientation, impairment of vision (cerebral oedema) (less frequent: hallucinations, spasms, comatose condition)
- nausea, emesia
- headache

Paraclinics:
- hyponatremia (▶ degrees of severity) and other electrolyte disorders (especially hypokaliaemia)
- Hb-decrease (hypervolemia)

- if necessary, haemolytic parameter
- disseminated intravascular coagulation (DIC)
- arterial blood gas analysis (BGA)

The extent of the fluid absorption can be estimated on the basis of serum sodium concentration and total extracellular fluid.

Equation:

Absorbed volume $= [(\text{pre Na}^+/\text{post Na}^+) \times \text{ECF}] - \text{ECF}$

- Absorbed volume: calculated amount of absorbed distending medium; pre Na^+: preoperative serum sodium concentration; post Na^+: postoperative serum sodium concentration; ECF: extracellular fluid, approximately $0.2 \times \text{kg}$ body weight

Reference:

Serocki G, Hanss R, Bauer M, Scholz J, Bein B: The gynecological TURP syndrome. Severe hyponatremia and pulmonary edema during hysteroscopy. Anästhesist 2009; 58: 30–4

Table 8.1: Degrees of severity of the TUR-syndrome.

	Na^+ (mmol/l)	Symptoms (overlapping)
slight	125–135	restlessness nausea emesis
medium	120–125	dyspnoea hypertonia/hypotonia cyanosis headache angina pectoris
severe	<120	CNS: increasing confusion, cerebral oedema kidney: oliguria, anuria lung: pulmonary oedema "resection shock": cardiac shock
	<110	unconsciousness, tetaniform spasms, **exitus**

(from: Lenz G, Kottler B, Schorer R, eds. MEMO-Anästhesie. Stuttgart: KE Verlag; 1985)

Forms of course of the TUR-syndrome:
- acute form:
- quick, mainly intravascular resorption of irrigation fluid with fast clinical symptoms through hypervolaemia and hyponatraemia
- late, "toxic" form:
- slow, mainly extravascular resorption out of the perimetran, perivesicular or peritoneal area with protracted clinical symptoms such as renal failure and ileus

Predisposing factors for the TUR-syndrome:
- large uterus (probe length >10 cm)
- myoma resection (especially with intramural myomas)
- high fluid deficit
- long duration of surgery
- multipara
- inexperienced surgeon

Therapy of the TUR-syndrome

General:
- termination of surgery
- insertion of bladder catheter
- control of in- and outflow
- fluid restriction

Hypervolaemia:
- loop diuretic (e.g. Furosemid)
- if necessary, osmotic diuretic

Plasma hypotonia (hyponatraemia):
- infusion of app. 1 l 1-molar sodium chloride solution (5.85%) from serum sodium concentration <125 mmol/l (quick)

Cardiac decompensation:
- increase of inotropism by dobutamine
- reduction of preload by nitroglycerine

Cerebral oedema:
- elevating the upper body
- if necessary, respiration with mild hyperventilation
- if necessary, glycocorticoids

Under therapy in progress:
- if necessary, tight control of serum electrolytes, arterial blood gas analysis, Hb-parameter, haemolytic parameter, serum osmolality

8.5 Burns

- very rare complication

Note: **Never** use an **electrolyte-containing** distending medium for electrosurgical **monopolar** hysteroscopy.

State-of-the-art electrosurgical instruments (Autocon 400) have different sensors warning the user of a possible risk for the patient. With the help of these sensors in combination with an automatic power adjustment, a maximum of safety in high-frequency surgery is reached. When older high-frequency instruments are used, severe burns near the neutral electrode may occur.

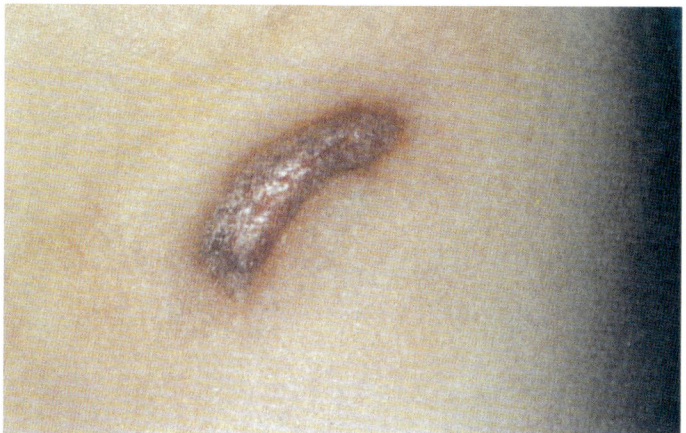

Fig. 8.5: Burn injury in the femoral region (position of the neutral electrode) as a result of electrosurgical surgery with electrolyte-containing distending medium (sodium chloride) and conventional high-frequency instrument.

8.6 Air embolism

- extremely rare complication

During operative hysteroscopy with a fluid distending medium an air embolism is theoretically possible.

Note: When resectates are removed by resectoscope with outer sheath in position, the resectoscope can only be re-inserted under constant supply of fluid.

Cave: Permanent intracavitary supply of air with opened vessels can cause air embolism.

Note: Watch that the supply tube does not contain air at the beginning of surgery as well as during the change of the bags containing the distending medium. If possible, planning of the amount of the distending medium before surgery to avoid changing the bags during surgery. (▶ page 16)

Clinical picture:
- signs of acute right ventricular load with vena cava superior syndrome
- decrease in blood pressure, tachycardia, arrhythmia
- possible: pulmonary oedema, hypoxaemia
- paradoxical arterial air embolism with open oval foramen with coronary ischaemia, ventricular fibrillation, neurological deficits
- increased dead space ventilation with quick decrease in final expiratory CO_2 partial pressure

Therapy:
- oxygen ventilation, turn off nitrous oxide
- PEEP-ventilation
- administration of sympathomimetic drugs
- administration of bronchodilating drugs (β_2- mimetics)

Presumed air embolism in a patient during a bipolar myoma resection with grade 2

TABELLAR TRENDS	6-MAI	6-MAI	6-MAI	6-MAI	6-MAI 2009 15:34
	14:50	14:55	15:00	15:05	15:10
HF	88	92	130	120	126
NBD-S	60	64	99		112
NBD-D	36	41	61		59
NBD-M	44	47	75		80
NBD-F	116	93	133		118
SPO2-%	94	57	82	99	100
SPO2-F	88	92	128	120	124
ST-I					
ST-II	0,5	-0,6	-0,6	-0,7	-0,7

Fig. 8.6: Decrease in O_2 saturation beginning at 14:50 o'clock (measured by pulse oyximetry, see SPO_2-%).
Note the simultaneously beginning change of the stoke trend in ECG (ST-II) indicating a continuing/persistent coronary ischaemia.

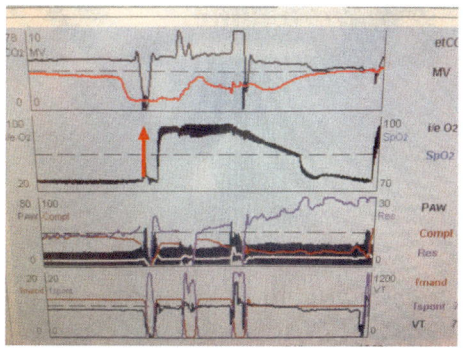

Fig. 8.7: Note the abrupt, transient slump of endtidal CO_2 in the anaesthetized patient – indicating to a short-term pulmo-arterial air embolism (see ↑).

Note: The risk of an air embolism is low although possible with the monopolar as well as the bipolar operation technique.

8.7 Frequency of complications

Table 8.2: Frequency of complications with different hysteroscopic surgeries.

	Perforation	Bleeding	TUR-syndrome (monopolar)	Infections
Myoma resection Grade 2	+ + +	+ + +	+ + +	+
Grade 0	+	+	+ +	+
Polyp resection	+	+	+	+
Endometrial ablation	+	∅	+	+
Endometrial resection	+ +	+	+ +	+
Septum dissection	+	+	+	+
Intrauterine adhesiolysis grades III/IV	+ + +	+	+ +	+

∅, no risk 0; +, low risk <1 %; + +, medium risk <5 %; + + +, increased risk >5 %

9 Special clinical cases

9.1 Hysteroscopic surgery of a hemihaematometra

Case report of a 14-year-old patient with cyclic lower abdominal pain on the right

Case history:
- appendectomy because of discomfort, performed externally by a surgeon
- laparoscopy performed externally, diagnosis: large intramural myoma on the right side
- referral for further therapy

Diagnostics:
- *speculum adjustment:* 1 portio
- *palpation:* uterus enlarged, extended to the right
- *sonography:* 10 cm solid structure with haematometra on the right

Therapy:
1. laparoscopy
2. operative hysteroscopy with incision of the right hemihaematometra (coagulum), irrigation of the right half of the cavity, tubal ostia visible on the right → insertion of IUD for 3 months
3. follow-up hysteroscopy after 3 months: regular uterine cavity with well proliferated endometrium

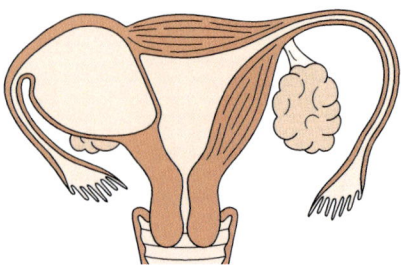

Fig. 9.1: Initial findings: hemihaematometra on the right.

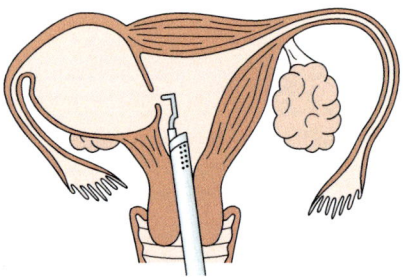

Fig. 9.2: Hysteroscopic incision of the hemihaematometra.

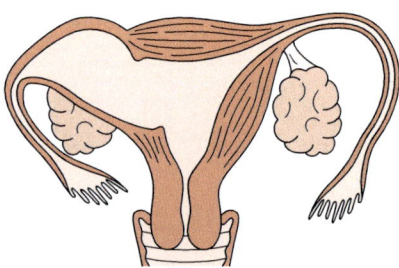

Fig. 9.3: Follow-up hysteroscopy: final findings after 3 months and after extraction of IUD.

9.2 Hysteroscopic resection of large residual placenta

Case report of a 24-year-old patient

state after partus with placenta accreta, afterwards 3 times hysteroscopy and abrasion, performed externally, both without success

Intraoperative:
- app. 7 cm "tumour" (placenta) well supplied with blood
- first surgery on 22 Jan 2006:
  bipolar resection of 214 g residual placenta (partly calcified)
- second surgery on 14 Feb 2006:
  bipolar resection of residual placenta

Conclusion:
Without bipolar resection removal is not possible (or only in many further interventions)

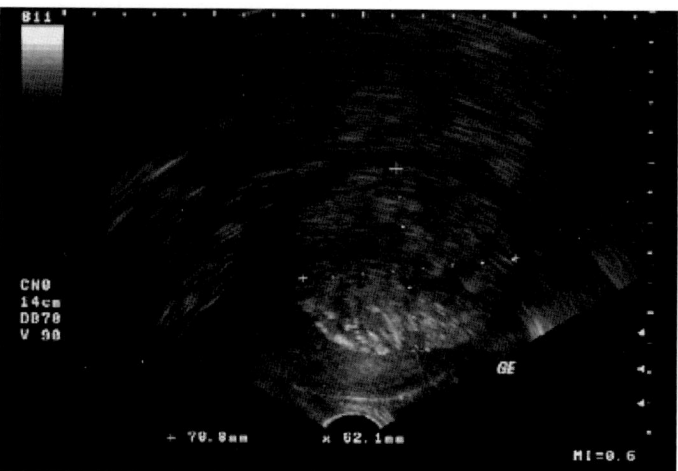

Fig. 9.4: Sonography – initial findings: large, highly vascularised residual placenta.

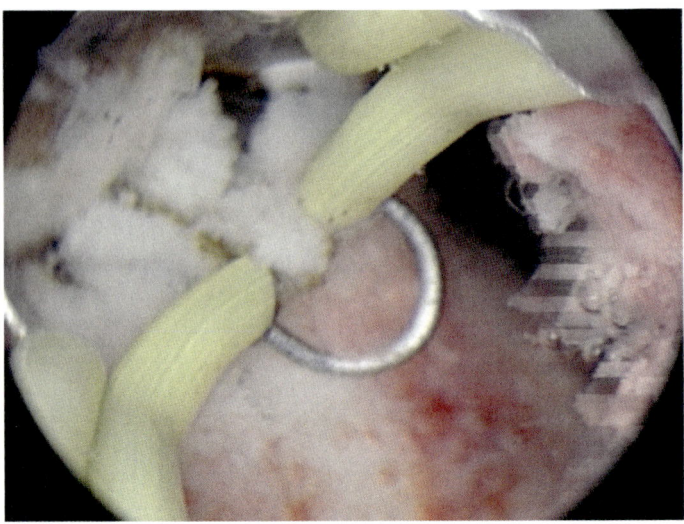

Fig. 9.5: Bipolar resection of the vascularised, partly calcified residual placenta.

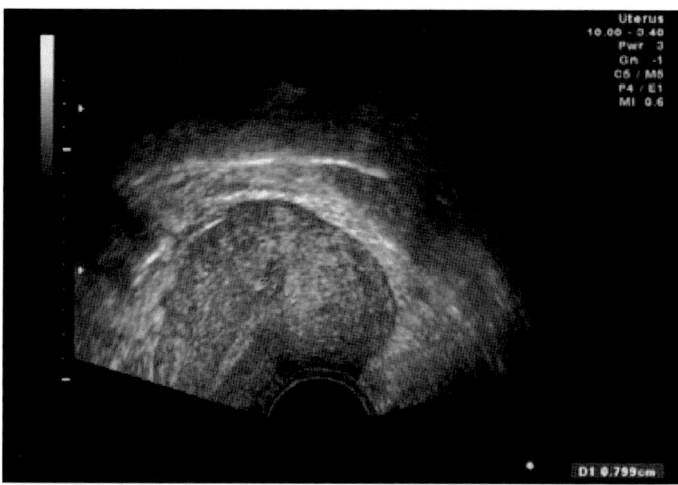

Fig. 9.6: Sonography – final findings after 3 months (regular uterine cavity), regular menstrual bleeding.

I thank Dr. Scheffler (Bremen) for the kind permission to use the sonographic images.

9.3 Myoma resection of a leiomyosarcoma

Case report of a 41-year-old patient

- recurrent menorrhagia for about 2 years

1. Sonography: 3 cm submucous-intramural myoma
2. Hysteroscopy: normal submucous myoma → myoma resection
3. Histology: leiomyosarcoma → hysterectomy + lymphadenectomy

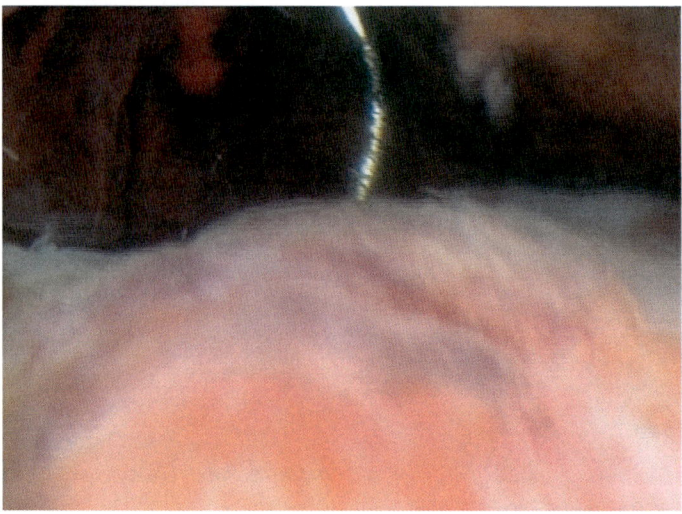

Fig. 9.7: Hysteroscopy: myoma without abnormalities; histology: leio-myosarcoma.

Note: Leiomyosarcomas are very rare and can be without findings in sonography and hysteroscopy.

Note: Therefore histological examinations of the myoma resectates are absolutely necessary. Vaporization methods (without histology) should be avoided.

10 Summary

Established indications for operative hysteroscopy:
- septum dissection in patients suffering from habitual abortions
- intrauterine adhesiolysis in infertile patients
- myoma resection of solitary submucous myomas in patients suffering from bleeding disorders and infertile patients
- endometrial ablation and -resection

Relative indications for operative hysteroscopy:
- septum dissection with primary and secondary infertility
- myoma resection of multiple myomas

With exact indications the operative hysteroscopy is an established minimally invasive method with excellent postoperative results and thus enriches the scope of operative gynaecology.

Note: The operative hysteroscopy has meanwhile become one of the standard gynaecological operations and should be part of the range of surgery in every hospital.

11 Further reading

Römer T: Diagnostic Hysteroscopy. A Practical Guide. 2nd edition.
  Berlin, New York: de Gruyter; 2010

Accompanying DVDs

Römer, Thomas
Operative Hysteroscopy
Media Service, Karl Storz GmbH, Tuttlingen
02/2005, order number KS 597

Römer, Thomas
Bipolar Technique for Intrauterine Surgery in Gynecology
Media Service, Karl Storz GmbH, Tuttlingen
09/2008, order number KS 699

e-mail: mediaservice@karlstorz.de

12 Index